THE LATEX ALLERGY CRISIS:
A FORGOTTEN EPIDEMIC

What Happened, Why it Happened, and What Happened to Me.
My Experience and the experience of others living with a Latex Allergy.

Margaret Konieczny RN, MSN

K and K Publishing
Carson City, NV 89721
Email: marge@kankpublishing.com
Webpage: http://kankpublishing.com/

ISBN   978-0-9828886-1-2

Copyright 2012

10 9 8 7 6 5 4 3 2 1

◊ "After the 3rd trip to ER with swollen eyes, itching, and tightness in my throat..."   —Denise

◊ "My eyes felt full, watery, and would tear all the time"—Marge

◊ "My hands were red, dry, cracked, and itchy; I began to wear latex gloves more often to hide my 'Hamburger Hands...'"   —Peg

◊ "I had to provide my own latex free gloves and I bought my own latex-free tourniquet..."   —Victoria

◊ "One day at the dentist my lip broke out in hives..."   —Pam

◊ "It is so frustrating to have other nurses' look at me in disbelief when I tell them I can't use a certain product due to my allergy."
                                                                            —Shari

◊ "Four hours after having protected sex with a latex condom, I had vaginal itching, redness and swelling."   — Anonymous

◊ "While assisting in surgery during a C-Section, my face swelled over my surgical mask. The anesthesiologist threatened to stop the C-Section if I didn't leave the room..."   —Traci

DISCLAIMER

This book is designed to bring information to the reader about how latex allergies became a crisis in the late 1980s. It is not the intention of the author to reprint all the material on the subject, but to explain what happened to her and to provide the interested reader with additional resources.

Every effort has been made to provide current and accurate information. This book should be used as a guide and not as the ultimate word on the subject of HIV/AIDS and the discovery of rubber.

The author and K and K Publishing shall have neither liability nor responsibility to any person or entity with respect to any loss or damage caused or alleged to have been caused, directly or indirectly, by the information contained in this book.

ACKNOWLEDGMENTS

John D. Saylor, MD FAAAP

Peggy Rourke-Nichols, RN MICN

Denise McCarthy

Victoria Powell RN

Mary Harper

Pam Waterman

Traci Hart, RN MSN

DEDICATION

This book was written so that others diagnosed with a latex allergy will feel validated, and for those who still have not yet identified their symptoms as a latex allergy, and to provide a source for healing.

INTRODUCTION

Articles have been written on the cause, symptoms, and treatments of latex allergy; however, there are few, if any, written experiences of those living with a hypersensitivity to latex. This book will cover my experience through early symptoms, diagnosis, Workers' Compensation issues and employer accommodations. The experiences of others living with a latex allergy are also included. There are several pictures in this book showing my anaphylactic reactions to latex. Viewers beware, these are not pretty, and I don't look happy.

Latex allergies affect the whole person, from the clothing they wear, foods they eat, places they visit, and their personal lifestyle. Their emotional as well as physical well being is affected. Latex allergies are permanent. There is no cure except strict avoidance, which is difficult to do; latex is ubiquitous.

In the 1980s people were dying from the newly identified, Human Immunodeficiency Virus (HIV). The virus spread through contact with infected blood and body fluids. The virus was not completely understood and, at first, it was causing fatal diseases in homosexual men. Later, hemophiliacs, needle drug users, and heterosexual men and women were presenting with the disease. As the death toll rose, fear and panic set in. In addition to HIV, hepatitis B was also becoming a significant health problem. Health care workers were at great risk of becoming infected with these viruses through needle sticks and dermal exposures to infected blood. By 1987, the Center for Disease Control (CDC) mandated that healthcare workers wear latex gloves when providing direct patient care. In 1988, the Occupational Safety and Health Administration (OSHA) joined with the CDC, in mandating *Standard Precautions*, the wearing of protective equipment, for all healthcare workers who are exposed to human blood and body fluids.

The incidence of latex allergies mushroomed with the increased use of latex gloves. By 1989, just two years after the CDC mandate, over 1,000 cases of latex allergy were reported including 15 deaths. The National Institute for Occupational Safety and Health (NIOSH) reported that since 1997 six percent of the general population and 18% of healthcare workers have become sensitized to latex proteins.

Reports of allergic contact dermatitis acquired from wearing rubber gloves were made as early as 1933 by Dr J.G. Downing. In his article, *Dermatitis from Rubber Gloves*, he indicates that glove manufacturers were aware of the allergic properties of latex proteins; however, there are over 60 different latex proteins. At the time, the glove manufacturers did not have the finances or expertise to determine which were the most allergenic.

Information about latex allergies came slowly and, by 1989, when the incidence of latex allergies had skyrocketed, physicians were unable to make definitive diagnoses of latex allergy and workers continued to be exposed to allergenic latex proteins.

The history of glove use in healthcare is surprisingly short. To those just entering the profession, it seems unbelievable that gloves and other personal protective equipment were not always worn by healthcare workers. As you will read, clean aseptic technique was not appreciated in the medical field until the late nineteenth century. Rubber glove use for surgical procedures did not occur until the late 1890s and was not accepted as routine until the 1920s.

It is imperative that today's healthcare professional be aware of latex as an allergen for themselves and for the care of their patients who are latex allergic. Health care facilities may still be using latex gloves, and the even more allergenic, powdered latex glove. Those who are already sensitized can, with continued exposure to latex, develop a serious hypersensitivity.

CONTENTS

FIGURES

Part I

Chapter 1

WHY NATURAL RUBBER LATEX GLOVES

Prior to 1983 glove use was limited to surgery, and in the performance of sterile procedures. Basic patient care was performed without gloves. What prompted the use of gloves in the routine daily care of patients was the identification of blood-borne viruses: first hepatitis B and then HIV.

Blood-borne Pathogens.

Being diagnosed with the HIV infection was considered a death sentence. This virus causes the disease AIDS (Acquired Immuno-deficiency Syndrome) for which there is no cure. In the mid 1980s this mysterious infection spread rapidly throughout the United States. It first gained attention in 1981 when 5 homosexual males in Los Angeles presented with a strange opportunistic pneumonia and a rare cancer. This was the overt beginning of the gay sexual liberation, when gay men and women struggled to openly express their sexual orientation. It is not known why the disease first manifested in the gay American male; however, the lifestyle and openness of gay men's sexual relationships at that time helped the disease to spread rapidly. By the end of 1981 five to six new cases were being reported each week. Information about the disease was practically non-existent. It was assumed the virus originated in Haiti and was brought to the United States by Haitian immigrants. Initially, it was believed to be spread only by sexually active gay men. By the end of 1983, new cases of AIDS were being diagnosed in epidemic proportions; of the 3,064 new cases, 1292 died.

In 1984, the virus was finally identified by French researchers. The virus was called lymphadenopathy-associated virus (LAV). Later it was changed to HIV. At the time there was no treatment. Fear and panic took hold among the gay community. The social stigma of being gay was now in the news more than ever before. People who acquired the disease were now known to be, or branded as, homosexual. "Coming out of the closet" was inevitable for gays when they presented with the disease. In 1985 a well-known movie star, Rock Hudson, who tried to keep his sexual orientation under cover, died of AIDS.

Soon it was discovered that hemophiliacs who received blood transfusions were being diagnosed with the disease. In 1986 it is estimated that half of the hemophiliacs in America had acquired the disease from infected blood. In addition, needle drug users who shared needles were also being diagnosed with AIDS. The phenomenon became known as the four "H" disease: Homosexuals, Hemophiliacs, Haitians and Heroin users. Once the routes of transmission were identified, the notion of it being only a gay man's disease was proved false. Today, heterosexual activity is the prime method of transmission in the world.

The HIV virus is a blood-borne pathogen. Any direct contact with infected blood by needle sticks, blood transfusions, donor organs, open sores or non-intact skin transfers the virus to the recipient. It is also transmitted to an unborn child from an infected mother through the Placenta. The virus is carried by semen and vaginal fluids and is transmitted with sexual activity. In 1985, the first government report acknowledging the disease was published. Believing the primary method of transmission was sexual contact, public sex education became top priority to stop the spread of the disease. It was discovered that the African chimpanzee carried a virus called Simian Immunodeficiency Virus (SIV). This virus was transmitted to humans and evolved into the human HIV strain. The mutated HIV virus was first identified in West Central Africa around 1959. African natives butchered monkeys for their meat. This practice is called bushmeat. The monkey virus was then transmitted to the native by bites or cuts in his hands during the slaughter. It is believed that the increased colonization of Africa by Europeans in the early 1900s, along with sexual promiscuity, rapidly spread the virus among the inhabitants. In addition, poor aseptic technique in administering immunizations to natives by reusing

2

contaminated needles contributed to the proliferation of the disease. Eventually, the virus traveled from Africa to Europe, Haiti, and to America. The United States was the first country to recognize the virus.

The virus attacks the human immune system. It suppresses the immune response against itself as well as other pathogenic (harmful) microorganisms. Infected people cannot fight off common infections.

At first they have frequent colds, flu's, and minor infections. As their immune system fails, opportunistic infections, pneumonias, and cancers occur. At this point, the contagion has progressed to the disease, AIDS. Two of the most devastating opportunistic infections for the AIDS patient are Pneumocystic carinii (now known as Pneumocystis jiroveci pneumonia), and Kaposi's sarcoma. Those afflicted became gravely ill, lost weight, and exhibited the wasting syndrome common with AIDS sufferers. They would generally die within five years of being infected, if not sooner.

Initially, treatment was non-existent. The first drug to combat AIDS was not discovered until 1987. With research, newer and better drugs have been discovered. These drugs are not a cure, but have proven to slow down the progression of the disease and prolong life expectancy. The best method of treatment is prevention.

Despite the global effort to educate people about the disease, AIDS has not been eradicated. Worldwide there are 40 million people living with HIV/AIDS. According to a United Nations report of November 2011, new cases of AIDS in the world have leveled off. The other good news is that deaths from AIDS have declined due to the new drug treatments available. In the most recent CDC report of 2009, it is estimated there were 48,100 newly diagnosed HIV infections in the United States. In July 2010, the CDC reported that there are approximately 1,106,400 people living with an HIV infection in the United States. (www.CDC.gov/hiv/topics/surveillance /incidents.htm). Due to the long window period, one out of five of those afflicted is not aware of his/her infection. The window period is the period between first exposure to the disease and until antibodies are developed and manifested in a blood test. This can take from months to years. During this time, infected individuals can transmit the virus to others.

The Glove Mandate.

Before the HIV virus was recognized, there was another, newly identified, blood-borne pathogen causing national alarm; hepatitis B, known by its initials, HBV. This virus attacks the liver and in time causes irreversible damage, resulting in serious, chronic liver disease and eventually liver failure. Not all infected people will have symptoms; however, they become carriers of the virus.

Because of these viruses, healthcare providers were at risk for contracting these diseases. In 1983, the Center for Disease Control (CDC) issued a report recommending a volunteer HBV vaccination program for healthcare providers. They also developed and published the first protocol for Blood and Body Fluid Precautions. This report *recommended* that the healthcare worker use gloves when coming in contact with blood *suspected to be infected with hepatitis B.*

Later, once the HIV virus was also identified and the epidemic incidence and fatal prognosis of the HIV infected person was acknowledged, the CDC, in 1985, revised the Blood and Body Fluid Precautions and called it Universal Blood and Body Fluid Precautions. Health care providers were to consider *all patients* to be potentially infectious for HIV, HBV, and other blood-borne pathogens. Gloves were to be worn when handling blood or bodily fluids such as spinal fluid, wound drainage, amniotic fluid, peritoneal fluid, semen, and vaginal fluids or any other bodily fluid visibly contaminated with blood. Body secretions such as feces, sputum, tears, urine and saliva were not considered harmful unless contaminated with blood. However, since blood is not always visible, gloves eventually were worn with all body fluid contact. In addition, if the healthcare provider had non-intact skin, open sores, or tiny cuts or lesions on their hands, they must wear gloves.

Universal Blood and Body Fluid Precautions meant every patient was assumed to be potentially infectious. Everyone, from babies to the elderly could be suspect. No one knew who might be carrying the HIV virus. The main purpose of wearing gloves was to protect the healthcare worker. Confidentiality laws and Patient Rights protected the patient from involuntary disclosure of his disease. There was fear among those afflicted with HIV that disclosure might cause discrimination and deny or restrict their care. The patient had to give written consent before being tested for the HIV antibody, and for disclosure. These laws were passed to assure the patient's anonymity and freedom from the stigma of having the disease.

The long window period complicated the problem even more. Not knowing who had the infection required the wearing of gloves for all patient contact. The patient could be a carrier of the virus and be infectious years before being diagnosed, and he or she may not even be aware of their own infectious state.

HIV antibody is a lab test and not a medical diagnosis. If the lab test was done prior to the patient's admission to the hospital, it would not necessarily be in the patient's chart. The medical diagnosis of AIDS is an approved diagnosis and could be listed on the chart as the patient's admitting diagnosis. But, for confidentiality purposes, the physician would choose another similar or alternate diagnosis; he could just write pneumonia.

For example, if a lab test measuring hemoglobin was done and it was low, the admitting diagnosis would be anemia, not low hemoglobin. A patient with a positive blood test for HIV, with no symptoms, could come into the hospital for an unrelated reason. The hospital staff would not know of his infectious state, therefore, to be safe, all patients had to be considered infectious.

In 1989 OSHA, the Occupational Safety and Health Administration joined the CDC in issuing guidelines for the prevention and transmission of HIV and HBV to healthcare and public safety workers. They renamed *Universal Precautions* to *Standard Precautions*. The new guidelines urged all healthcare employers to provide work practice controls to minimize the worker's risk. These controls included providing personal protective equipment: gloves, masks, gowns, and eye wear. Hazardous material protocols were to be established for the handling of contaminated materials and linens. Needle and sharp disposal procedures were outlined and required. The procedures for handling used needles and sharps included no recapping of needles, placement of needle disposal boxes in each patient room, and correct labeling of contaminated items. Employers were to provide education and training, and medical follow-up for any exposure incidents.

Non-sterile, powdered natural rubber latex gloves were believed to be the best material to provide an adequate barrier between infectious pathogens and the wearer of the glove. The wearing of gloves and changing them before and after each patient became the best method to prevent the transmission of any infectious disease to the healthcare worker as well as to other patients. It took months to retrain the nurses and to make glove wearing a habit.

Some of the reasons for not wearing gloves were: too time consuming, loss of tactile feel, waste of gloves, gloves not in a convenient place, *"I've always used bare hands"* or just *"I forgot"*. Hand washing also increased. Patients at first seemed offended when the nurse wore gloves. They thought the nurses considered them infected with the HIV/AIDS. Eventually they realized the gloves protected them too. In fact, the patients became very astute in reminding the caregivers to wash their hands before and after touching them and to wear gloves.

If a healthcare worker was exposed to blood, and especially by needle stick, the patient was asked to submit to a HIV antibody blood test. The patient had to give their written consent for the blood test. Maintaining confidentiality, the patient, his doctor, and the involved healthcare worker, would be the only ones to know the results. Most patients consented. Even if the test was negative, it did not mean the patient was virus free. As stated before, it takes months to years for the virus antibody to be evident in a lab test. During this time the virus is growing and the carrier is infectious to others. This was an especially scary time for medical professionals. Some of my nurse colleagues refused to care for homosexual patients or any patient with suspected or related diagnoses.

At my hospital an interesting event happened. A surgeon cut through his glove and his finger with a scalpel while performing an appendectomy. The doctor bandaged his bleeding finger, changed his gloves and continued with surgery. When the patient was awake and was told what had happened, he was asked to give his consent to be tested for HIV. The patient agreed, but also insisted the surgeon be tested too, a reasonable but surprising request. If the surgeon's finger bled while cutting through the patient's abdomen, and the surgeon had a HIV infection, he could be transmitting the disease to the patient. Coincidently, confidentiality laws do not require a healthcare worker with an HIV infection to reveal it. As a matter of fact, in 1988, of the 61,929 cases of HIV/AIDS reported to the CDC, 5.1% were healthcare workers (MMWR Vol. 38, No. S-6 1989).

Chapter 2

MY STORY

In 1990, I was working as a hospital staff nurse. My hands were constantly red, rough, and dry. The skin would split around the nails and tips of my fingers. A red, itchy, rash covered both hands. It appeared to be a severe case of chapped hands from frequent hand washing. Over the next year, it was not only persistent, but became progressively worse. In addition to my hands all of my skin was extremely dry. By 1991, in addition to the persistent dermatitis and dry skin, my face was puffy, swollen and red. My eyes watered all the time; the eyelids were puffy, red and itchy. Slowly the dermatitis spread to my neck and shoulders. The itching was intense especially at night. The more I scratched, the more I damaged the skin. It was difficult to sleep. I would lie awake scratching one itchy, prickly area with some relief when another area started to tingle. It was maddening!

My face became so irritated I quit using soaps and astringents on my face. I looked prematurely older because of the puffy, dry, burgundy skin around my eyes.

Visine eye drops were a constant item in my purse. I used every type of Visine they made. Nothing helped for long; the feeling of fullness in my eyes was constant.

All this time, I thought it was hay fever, pollen allergies, and just plain extremely dry skin. I had eczema as a child and I thought it was recurring. I did not relate my symptoms to the increased use of latex gloves at work. However, when I was away from work, the rash and itching would subside. I attributed this to the fact that I did not wash my hands as often and I was able to keep the hand cream from being constantly washed off.

From 1992 to 1998 there was a slow, persistent progression of symptoms. Eventually the rash, redness, swelling, burning and itching covered my entire body (see Figure 1). By the time I was correctly diagnosed in 1998 my symptoms included angioedema (total body edema) and bronchial asthma. I became physically, mentally, and emotionally drained.

As you will see, my struggle during this time was due largely to the lack of information about latex allergies, and the medical community's lack of knowledge or acceptance of the problem.

Back in 1991, the first doctor I saw was my own primary care physician. We explored all the possibilities of seasonal allergies and reoccurring eczema. He prescribed hydrocortisone creams and antihistamines. With no lasting relief, he recommended a dermatologist.

In 1992 I started seeing a dermatologist who prescribed all the routine therapies; increasing the strength of cortisone creams; trials of different antihistamines, oils and lotions. Because of my blotchy facial redness, he performed a biopsy skin test for discoid erythematous lupus plus a lupus blood test. One of the physical signs of lupus is a blotchy red butterfly facial mask and a scaly red rash. He wanted to rule lupus out. He did, the tests came back negative.

He prescribed weekly ultraviolet light treatments, and tar baths which are used for eczematous and psoriasitic conditions. The ultraviolet light did little to improve the skin condition. The tar baths seemed to make things worse. The bath water was black and oily with an oily smell. My skin became redder and dryer after each bath and the itching increased. These are common side effects of coal tar. It has a large chemical composition which possibly could be related to the chemicals used in latex production. At this time there was some information surfacing about the possibility of healthcare workers having allergic reactions to latex gloves. When I questioned the dermatologist about this he did not agree and brushed it aside. He was focused on my history of atopic eczema and allergies as a child. Since there still wasn't enough information on the subject of latex allergy I went along with his assumptions.

While I was seeing the dermatologist I went to see an ophthalmologist for my watery, itchy eyes. He had no comment on the etiology (cause) of the symptoms. He was focused on my past history of allergies and did agree that I had a severe allergic optic response. He prescribed a new eye drop called Opticrom, a Cromolyn Sodium solution. It was so new a local pharmacist had to mix the formula. He also prescribed a cortisone eye ointment for temporary use. For a time it was a great relief! My eyes felt almost normal again.

In September 1993, with no permanent improvement, a friend suggested that I see a physician who specialized in holistic therapies for allergies. I entered into the ELISA/ACT program, which used measures intended to help the patient rebuild his immune system by changes in diet and lifestyle. Hypnosis and biofeedback was a part of the treatment. I tried it all with no lasting relief.

This holistic physician suggested an extensive analysis of the digestive tract and the ELISA/ACT blood test which was done in October 1993. The results indicated that I had a mild digestive problem with foreign bacteria in the GI tract. I was started on a therapeutic regime of antibiotics and then an intestinal flora replacement drug. It was also indicated that I had allergies to twenty-six different foods with some mild and intermediate reactions. What is interesting is that I never ate some of these foods before such as parsnips and sardines. We continued with the belief that the newly identified allergens were the culprit.

I removed all suspect foods from my diet. I clarified butter, made bread from sourdough starter as I was supposedly allergic to yeasts. I stopped using hydrogenated oils and avoided all the foods which I had some allergic response to. Once the foods were eliminated they could be reintroduced into the diet one by one to identify them as the current offending allergen.

I followed the regime. My symptoms continued. I was frustrated and disappointed. I requested a two week sick leave around the first of November 1993. During that time, I had some relief of symptoms. However, after going back to work in December my symptoms returned.

I began to feel a great deal of stress regarding the eczema, the itching, and my overall physical appearance. I requested, and my physician recommended, a three month medical leave of absence. He assumed workplace stress was causing the exacerbations of eczema. He was becoming as frustrated as I was and he abandoned the holistic methods and prescribed the following medications: Periactin for itching, Claritin for an antihistamine, Xanax and Zoloft for my stress and depression, and a histamine 2 blocker, Tagamet. In addition, I continued to avoid the foods I was deemed allergic to. Finally by January 31, 1994, being off work for approx six weeks, I began to feel better and the symptoms disappeared. By March 7th I was back at work and shortly after I returned, the symptoms reappeared. Yet, still no positive connection was made between the use of latex gloves and my reactions. I, however, had an underlying suspicion that latex gloves were the problem.

In 1993, *The Boston Globe* reported mysterious allergies were occurring among the Brigham and Women's Hospital operating room employees. Their symptoms were rashes, hives, respiratory irritation and nausea. They labeled it a "sick building syndrome." After an investigation, it was determined to be allergic reactions to latex gloves and other latex equipment. It was further determined that the cornstarch powder in the glove aerosolized the latex proteins which would electrostatically adhere to environmental surfaces. That same year, the Mayo Clinic announced that latex glove proteins were allergenic. They began a search for gloves that were labeled hypoallergenic for their staff (Edlich, 1997). Later in 1997, the FDA determined that the label of hypoallergenic was misleading, and ordered the glove manufacturers to remove the label from their boxes.

My employer began providing vinyl gloves as an alternative; however, powdered latex gloves were still being used in the facility. Unbeknownst to us at the time, the powder was a major route of spreading the latex proteins in the air. Recklessly snapping off gloves and pitching them into a wastebasket was a common occurrence. We now know minute particles of cornstarch, laden with latex proteins, become airborne by this action and can be inhaled. In addition, the cornstarch particles, combined with the latex proteins, could land on other surfaces and be picked up by clothing or touch.

I continued to see my primary physician and the dermatologist. Through 1994, '95 and '96 my symptoms decreased with each vacation or absence from work only to return when I went back. I continued to use lots of moisturizing creams and lotions; hydrocortisone creams, Opticrom eye drops, and all the different Visine types, Periactin, Tagamet, antihistamines, and the antidepressant Zoloft.

I felt lost. I couldn't figure out what was happening. Was it stress? Was it seasonal allergies? Was it work related? Some days were better than others and I just dealt with it. It wasn't totally interfering with my life. I was a single mother and nursing was my life. I loved it. I couldn't think of anything else that I wanted to do, and besides, I needed to work.

Around this time, the hospital started twelve hour shifts. I would work three days and be off four. That schedule seemed to ease the reactions. My lifelong dream was to teach nursing. I thought that would be a good way to end my career in nursing and to limit my exposure to the hospital environment. Since I was unsure if my work environment was the cause of my allergic reactions and skin problems, a change of venue was at least some course of action. Online courses now made it possible for students in rural areas, like me, to earn college degrees. So in 1995 I began to study for my MSN degree.

In the spring of 1997, ten years after CDC mandated universal blood and body fluid precautions, the National Institute for Occupational Safety and Health (NIOSH) posted an alert bulletin for employers. It was titled, *Preventing Allergic Reactions to Natural Rubber Latex in the Workplace*. It began with a warning:

> **"Workers exposed to latex gloves and other products containing natural rubber latex may develop allergic reactions such as skin rashes; hives, nasal, eye, or sinus problems; asthma and (rarely) shock."**

NIOSH recommended healthcare facilities train and educate workers on appropriate work practices, substitute non-latex products when appropriate, and monitor worker symptoms of latex allergy. In November 1997 my employer began to follow the mandate. They began to identify and eliminate latex items in the healthcare facility. Employees were educated on the health hazards of latex, how to identify allergy symptoms, and to use non-latex gloves if symptoms occur.

Many medical supplies were identified as containing latex. Most in themselves do not create a health problem. But with repeated exposure, and the increase use of powdered natural rubber latex gloves, sensitivities developed. The incidence of glove use went from 785 million in 1980 to 9.5 billion in 1995 (Gehring and Ring, 2000). Once sensitized, the individual has to avoid all latex products, which is a difficult task. Latex, as an important commodity, is everywhere. It can be found in more than 40,000 products from clothing, bedding, kitchen utensils, cleaning gloves, baby bottle nipples, and condoms.

There followed an explosion of information about latex allergies. In the December 1997 issue of the Annuals of Allergy, Asthma and Immunology, the American College of Allergy, Asthma and Immunology (ACAAI) submitted a joint subcommittee statement with American Academy of Allergy, Asthma, and Immunology (AAAAI), which states, in part:

> **IgE mediated latex allergy is the result of the exposure of susceptible individuals to latex rubber proteins. Medical devices particularly latex gloves are the largest single source of exposure to these potent allergens. Exposure may be by direct contact or by inhalation of allergen carried by cornstarch powder with which most latex gloves are coated. The clinical manifestations of latex allergy range from mild contact urticaria to anaphylaxis (p. 487).**

In October 1997, with this new information, my primary physician ordered a new blood test for latex hypersensitivity called, *IBT latex specific IgE panel*. The normal buffered latex count is below 5. My results were way above normal: my buffered latex count was 170 and glove latex extract count twenty. The results were definitive. He was so surprised that he took the time to call me at home. Finally there it was: proof of my allergic response to latex.

He advised that I avoid latex in my work environment, although he did not write out a work release. He also stated that his office did not file insurance claims with Workers' Compensation insurance companies. Since work release papers were not submitted to the hospital, I continued to work. I was not sure what I was looking for at this time. Discovering that I had an elevated IgE proved I had a latex allergy. What should I be doing about it? I did not get any direction from my physician. Since he did not work with Workers' Compensation insurance, it felt like he was done with it. At work I avoided latex as much as possible, yet I was still having problems. The hospital was trying to eliminate latex items, but the process was slow and sporadic. At this time non-latex nitrile gloves were becoming available.

My employer slowly replaced all latex patient care items. In some departments, however, such as surgery, powdered latex gloves were still being used. The surgeons preferred the latex glove for strength and feel. At the time it was not appreciated that cornstarch powder, laden with latex proteins, became airborne, and adhered to ventilation system filters. If not changed, the tainted air is circulated throughout the building. All employees are breathing the aerosolized powder over and over again and in all areas of the hospital.

Over the next few months I made several trips to the Emergency Room (ER) with exacerbation of symptoms. On February 18, 1998 I went to the ER for another severe flare-up of facial swelling, angioedema, itchy, red, watery eyes, and excoriations on my face, neck, shoulders and body. My skin was inflamed and it felt stressed and irritated. There was a constant burning, stinging and itching; and a feeling of unrest. The skin was in a tender, vulnerable state and, scratched, easily damaged. This time I was given a Kenalog (corticosteroid) injection and was told by the ER physician to fill out a Workers' Compensation Claim and to follow-up with the hospital's employee occupational health department.

I followed up with the occupational health nurse and she recommended that I see an allergist. My primary care physician also suggested I see an allergist in Reno, Nevada.

The year 1998 brought more information about latex allergy from federal organizations. The National Institute for Occupational Safety and Health (NIOSH) funded a grant for occupational safety and health research. The purpose was to study occupational injuries and illnesses and their underlying causes. The Food and Drug Administration (FDA) and a panel of experts telecasted a video conference on natural rubber latex allergy in February of 1998.

The first time I met the allergist he informed me he did not file claims or interact with Workers' Compensation Insurances either. I still didn't know enough about Workers' Compensation to know what my rights were. I just hoped he would give my employer and me some direction on how to deal with my problem. I knew I needed to get out of the hospital environment. Surprisingly, he said he didn't think my reactions were due to a latex allergy. I thought, *"What? Doesn't he have any information about latex allergy?"* I felt dejected, but with no other recourse, I consented to his allergy skin testing. He proceeded to test me for all the common allergens and included latex. At this time, there was no reliable skin test (and still isn't) for latex allergy. He devised his own test solution by placing a piece of a latex glove in sterile saline and then performed a skin prick test with the solution. He also taped a piece of a latex glove to my back for four days. The reaction to all of the skin tests was weak to moderate. He stated the latex tests were inconclusive. The testing did indicate I was allergic to phenylenediamine, which we now know is one of the chemicals used in processing rubber and manufacturing Spandex. He was reluctant to diagnose a latex allergy, even with the elevated IgE. After the testing he sent a follow-up letter to my primary physician stating his diagnosis *"Atopic Dermatitis possible contact Dermatitis ... and the significance of latex contact in causing her skin problems is currently not definably known."*

I felt alone and lost. There were times I began to doubt myself. *"Why weren't these physicians willing to learn about latex allergy and help me out?"*

During the allergy testing my symptoms worsened as I was told not to use any antihistamines. I looked and felt bad but it didn't matter. I needed to be antihistamine free in order to get accurate testing results. My skin condition became so severe the allergist gave me a two week work release due to "severe eczema."

I felt my work relationship was getting pretty strained at this time. I had been off work numerous times in the past few years because of the reactions. No one said anything to me directly, but I could feel their frustration with me when I brought in a work release note. The nursing manager had to find a replacement for me each time. That puts a strain on all the staff. I felt that administration wasn't going to do anything to help me until I had a definite diagnosis. Once I filed a Workers' Compensation claim I felt like an outsider among my colleagues and management, even if they were my friends, who wouldn't discuss it. I had the burden of proof for my work-related injury.

Again, after two weeks off my skin improved. The week before I returned to work, I bought a new bathing suit and went on a weekend trip. One hour after wearing the bathing suit in a swimming pool, I began to itch. By morning, all of my symptoms returned. That was the first time I realized Spandex could cause the same type of reactions. Two primary causes of latex sensitivities are the latex proteins themselves and the chemicals added to latex in the manufacturing process. Spandex is a synthetic fiber without latex proteins. However, chemicals are added to the fibers during the finishing processes. Many people already sensitized to chemicals used in latex manufacturing may develop dermatitis from Spandex garments. Also, many swimsuits have latex rubber elastic in the leg bands and/or straps. I used to think Lycra was different from Spandex. It is not. Lycra is the trade name.

When I presented myself to the allergist the following Monday he finally acknowledged that my reactions could be due to latex and Spandex in the

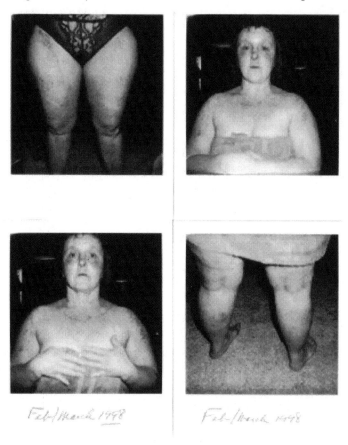

Feb/March 1998   Feb/March 1998

Figure 1. Angioedema, April 1998
Copyright 2012, Margaret Konieczny.

bathing suit. However, he stated I could go back to work at the hospital, avoid latex contact, and use non latex vinyl gloves for my job.

After I returned to work on April 23, 1998 my symptoms again reappeared, this time quickly and with increased intensity (see Figure 1). I had angioedema: total body swelling. My knees were so swollen I could feel the fullness of my skin behind my knees when I walked. The rash was everywhere.

I was feeling short of breath and miserable. Here I am again, without any support from the physician or my employer. I remember the first day back to work the nursing supervisor looked at me in disbelief and with sympathy but offered no remedy. I felt alone.

I needed to work. I felt frustrated and scared. I couldn't get anyone to help me out and tell me what to do. I had to figure this out on my own. I decided to transfer to an available home health position at my current employer.

This department had its office outside of the hospital building. That would be perfect for me, plus, patient care is done in the patient's home. I would be working in a latex-safe environment and I could have more control of the environment to make it latex safe for me. I applied for that position on April 23, 1998. I was not granted the transfer. The position was given to a colleague and friend of mine, I believed, because of all my absences from work. The director of the home health department didn't want to take on my problems including my many possible absences.

Again feeling frustrated, like I didn't matter and with no other place to go, I continued to work in the hospital. One of my colleagues suggested I search the internet for a physician. Surfing the internet was a giant leap for me. I was familiar with computers but the internet was overwhelming. It was a very new entity of information in 1998. I was somewhat skeptical. However, I typed in the search box *latex allergy* and what I found changed my life.

Finding a Physician Who Knows.

The web site for Allergy to Latex Education and Resource Team (ALERT), now called the American Latex Allergy Association (ALAA) popped up on my computer screen. This group was sponsoring legislation to prohibit the use of powdered latex gloves in healthcare institutions. Their mission was and is to increase national awareness of latex allergy and to provide information and give support to latex allergic individuals.

I emailed the organization and asked if they knew of any physicians in my area, Reno to Sacramento, who was knowledgeable about latex allergies. I was surprised to get a quick response. They provided me with a list of allergists and one of them on the list was Dr. John Saylor in Sacramento, California.

Help at last. I saw him on May 1, 1998. He took one look at me, listened to my story and he understood. After all I had been through; I was surprised that he had no doubt about my diagnosis and promptly stated my condition was due to latex exposure. He did not hem and haw. He knew! I sat there with an overwhelming sense of amazement. After all these years, I finally felt validated. I felt someone cared and listened to me. I felt like the chain I had been dragging was cut off.

He told me he was well acquainted with latex allergy individuals. He was the physician consultant for Sacramento-region Sutter Hospital regarding latex allergies. He also was familiar with Workers' Compensation insurance laws and knew the correct procedure for filing a claim in California.

The initial office visit with Dr. Saylor lasted three hours. I had a physical exam and a Pulmonary Function Test (PFT). Dr. Saylor concluded that I had a latex allergy due to prolonged exposure to latex in my work environment. He spent the rest of the time talking to me and reviewing the cause, the signs and symptoms, and the prognosis of latex allergy. He prescribed an appropriate drug regime.

Dr. Saylor explained the process of filing for Workers' Compensation. He knew the language, and he wrote the appropriately worded work release stating; "*She is unable to return to work until a latex-safe environment was provided. Occupational Injury Report to follow.*" On the report, he wrote the following diagnosis, "*Asthma due to occupational latex exposure for more than 5 years and occupational eczema due to latex exposure.*" My life changed almost immediately.

Chapter 3

LIFE AFTER DIAGNOSIS

Employer's Response

I presented Dr. Saylor's note to the Director of the Personnel Department. I was immediately put on medical leave. He told me to go home and he would contact me in a few days. After a few days, may be a week (I really don't recall the length of time) he called and told me they were transferring me to the home health department and I was to start in one week. He also told me the nursing director wanted to fire me. Fear ran through me when he said *"fire me."* This is the first time I felt any animosity from my employer. I don't think I heard him say anything else until he said, "I advised her against it." I understand now that firing me would have greater consequences for the hospital since I had filed a Workers' Compensation claim. When I got off the phone, I was feeling worried but relieved that Dr. Saylor's correctly worded documents made a difference. All this time, I did not get angry or complain about my employer to other employees. I am not the type to be that vocal. I never discussed the details of my situation with anyone except my family because I didn't want to cause any trouble. I liked working for this hospital and I needed to work. I believe that behavior was to my advantage. I just did what I needed to do to take care of myself. All I wanted is to get out of the hospital environment, continue to work, and for someone to believe me.

I began my first day in the home health department on May 24th 1998. I felt some uneasiness in the home health office. I knew there was a lot of discussion behind my back about my transfer. I did not know what they were saying. I had a feeling the home health director did not like being forced to give me a position and create a new job category for me. But she did. I was now the new home health Aide Coordinator. This position kept me in the office and I would not have any patient contact. I was ecstatic, smug, and cautious. I did not talk to anyone about the process of getting the position. I went about my job as professionally as I could. I kept the comment about firing me to myself.

I made my environment as latex free as possible. I removed rubber bands, used latex-free pencil erasers, bought my own latex-free blood pressure cuff and did not lick envelopes. The glue used on envelopes has a latex base. I had my own box of nitrile gloves and I was not required to make home care visits at this time.

Healing.

Now that I was internet savvy, I continued to use the internet to search for more information. Latex allergy was in the news now. Because of my research, I made changes to my clothing. I no longer wore pantyhose or knee high stockings. Luckily, bare legs were beginning to be the fashion again. I purchased latex-free undergarments and avoided any clothing with elastics or with Spandex fibers.

I was healing. It was a slow process. Dr. Saylor's prescribed drug regime initially included prednisone, an oral corticosteroid, for a specified length of time. He prescribed a daily antihistamine and a histamine two blocker like Pepcid. For itching at night, he prescribed Hydroxyzine (Vistaril), and added Doxipen for severe nighttime burning and itching. Once the itching was under control, I stopped the Doxipen and continued the Vistaril until the itching totally subsided. At that point, Vistaril would be on an "as needed" basis. I considered Vistaril to be a miracle drug for me. Vistaril is a CNS depressant and a mild sedative. Its therapeutic effects include decreasing the effects of histamine, especially pruritis (itching). Doxipen is an antianxiety agent and also has antihistamine properties. Finally, I could sleep through the night. What a relief. I felt human again. My skin and appearance improved along with my self-esteem.

I began to realize my hypersensitivity to latex was not restricted to my work environment. It affected every part of my life. Now healed, and out of the hospital, other types of non-industrial latex exposure became evident. Foods I had always been able to eat in the past were creating allergic reactions. The first was bananas. In August I ate one of my favorite desserts, bananas and ice cream. Within twelve hours my face began to swell and sting, I had generalized itching, and a flushed face and neck. The sting changed to a burning sensation. The rash reappeared. I used cold compresses and the usual medications. Nothing would stop it. Once the reaction started it had to run its course. Medications only helped alleviate the symptoms. This reaction required a visit to the allergist who put me on another round of prednisone.

As the time went on, I discovered I was allergic to avocados, kiwi, and mangos as well.

The next exposure I had was to the everyday product, Johnson & Johnson Band Aids. I used a Band Aid to cover a cut on my finger and by morning my finger and hand was swollen, red and itchy. I had not realized the Band Aid adhesive was latex based. I added Band Aids to my list of things to avoid. Johnson and Johnson did not manufacture a latex free product. I searched and found several latex-free bandages made by other companies.

At home, I continued my vigilance and maintained my home environment as latex-free as possible. All my healthcare providers were alerted. My dentist was very accommodating. I always was the first patient of the day. He and his staff always used latex-free items around me. When I had knee surgery I was the first case of the day. Even though the hospital tried to be as latex-safe as possible, I had a reaction. After surgery, in the recovery room, my face began to itch. In my semi-awake state, I kept pulling off the oxygen mask; the nurses kept putting it back on. The next day my face was red and swollen (see Figure 2). I notified the hospital of my reaction and it was discovered the elastic on the mask was latex.

I continued to do well, and I was healing and happy in my new position in home health. Soon I would learn of the Workers' Compensation process and its value. In retrospect, I can see how the events and decisions of the past influenced the future.

Workers' Compensation.

On June 4, 1998, four months after filing my claim, I received a letter from the hospital's Workers' Compensation insurance company, Risk Manage-

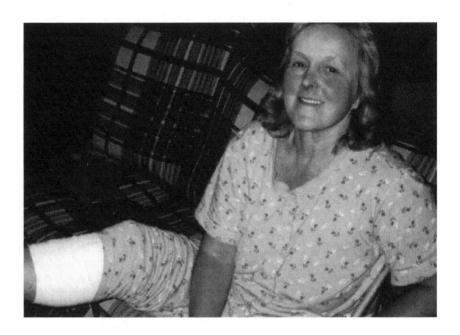

Figure 2. Post-surgery. Copyright 2012, Margaret Konieczny.

ment. The claims adjuster wrote that the hospital accepted my claim and the insurance company would pay off my related doctor bills. They would reimburse the state of California for any state disability payments I received (While on medical leave I did not have enough compensated sick time, so I filed for state disability.). I was to forward any documentation and bills regarding my claim. Great! I was happy to have this resolved. In August, when I had that reaction after eating bananas, I needed a physician visit.

The insurance carrier, Risk Management, considered this exposure a non-industrial event. They did not want to pay for the office visit.

Traditionally, Workers' Compensation covers "on the job" injuries. However, an industrially caused latex allergy has implications in every part of our lives. Latex is used in millions of products outside of the hospital environment.

It would take some time before the Risk Management Company would understand latex allergy. Physician documents had to be sent explaining the ramifications of latex in the environment and cross-reactive foods which also cause similar reactions in latex sensitive individuals.

From August 1998 until March 2000, the communication with the insurance adjuster was infrequent, sometimes frustrating, and often confusing. I do not recall all the conversations. He talked about compensation rates, my rights and responsibilities, and tried to have me agree to sign off the claim. I didn't understand the Worker Compensation codes he mentioned. He would send me some information from time to time.

I continued my research on latex allergies and identified other latex items in my environment that may cause a reaction. One of them was balloons. Rubber balloons have a powder coating to keep them from sticking together. If a balloon breaks, the powder scatters the latex proteins in the air. I avoid all areas with latex balloons.

I continued to see Dr. Saylor for follow-up visits. By March 1999 I was managing, and able to control, my sporadic reactions with the prescribed drug therapy and learning to avoid latex exposures.

Over the next year, Dr. Saylor sent progress reports to the Risk Management Company. In February 2000, in response to a Risk Management inquiry, he wrote; *"according to the California Code and Regulations Title 8 Section 9785 this patient is "Permanent and Stable."* He stated I would require lifetime medical care as I had a *"permanent immunological disorder."* In addition in a note to me and the insurance company he wrote:

"There is hidden latex in the environment and with each exposure she may have an immediate and severe return of symptoms and risk further permanent increase in the degree of sensitivity. She could return to work only if it is a latex-safe environment."

This is where physician knowledge of industrial injuries and Workers' Compensation laws is worth their weight in gold. With that last statement from Dr. Saylor, I began to have some serious conversations with the claims adjuster, and on March 2000 I received a Notice Regarding Permanent Disability benefits from Risk Management.

In the report it stated that I would begin to receive disability payments at fifteen percent of my current rate of pay. In addition, Dr. Saylor's report of "Permanent and Stable" would be sent to the State Disability Division of the Department of Industrial Relations for their disability rating.

Workers' Compensation settlements are based on predetermined disability codes and ratings. Ratings are expressed in percentages of how much of your job you cannot perform. For instance, there is a certain rating for loss of limb, loss of sight, etc. In addition, the rating is determined by the date of injury, your age, and occupation and diminished future earnings.

Since latex allergy at the time was not considered a disability, it did not have its own disability code in California. On April 17, 2000, the California Department of Industrial Relations finally made a Summary Rating Determination based on "dermatological condition resulting in strict avoidance of contact with latex." However, the determination stated "future medical treatment required" and the Permanent Rating Disability is twelve percent. Based on this my compensation was lowered.

In May 2000 the claims adjuster indicated I might be eligible for Vocational Rehabilitation. I immediately assumed I might qualify for tuition reimbursement for my Master's Degree since I was "rehabbing" myself. Dr. Saylor had indicated that I was a Qualified Injured Worker (QIW). I learned that according to California State Workers' Compensation Law, if the employer is unable to provide the worker with a safe working environment then the worker qualifies for Vocational Rehabilitation.

However, I was informed by the claims adjuster that since I was transferred to home health, a latex safe environment, the hospital had provided me with a latex safe environment. So, I no longer qualified for Vocational Rehabilitation.

In July 2000, I was informed by the claims adjuster that my disability payments had ended. At this point he began to talk about settlements and encouraged me to sign off my claim. He became pushy and rude. He again quoted Worker Compensation codes which I didn't understand. He stated that since my condition had improved, I could sign off my claim. He said I had received the max in compensation. Something didn't feel right. I kept telling him I wasn't expecting any monetary compensation. All I wanted was medical coverage for the rest of my life for an injury that is permanent. At that point I wasn't getting good answers from him.

In retrospect, if they had accepted me into the home health department when I applied for the position back in April 1998 I am sure there wouldn't have been any further action taken on my part. I was pursuing a remedy all on my own. I intended to finish my degrees and teach nursing. More importantly, I didn't want to create any animosity with my employer. I needed them so that I could continue to work and pay for my education.

On July 7, 2000, the claims adjuster wanted me to sign a "Compromise and Release" which would release all issues, future medical care, and right to re-open my case, for a total settlement of $5,355. Now I understood what he was trying to do and I saw the implications. I kept reiterating my need for future medical coverage but it was obvious we would not come to an agreement. At this point I realized I needed a lawyer who specialized in Workers' Compensation Law.

Finding a Lawyer.

After contacting several lawyers in my hometown, none would take my case. I again emailed the support group ALERT and asked if they knew of a lawyer in my vicinity who was knowledgeable about latex allergy and occupational injury. I received a list of names. The first law office on the list couldn't take my case as they were already involved in a suit with the manufacturers of latex gloves. They did refer me to another law firm in Oakland, California. On August 7th 2000, the law office of Boxer & Gerson, LLP took my case. All conversations were now between the insurance claims adjuster and my lawyer. I was advised to not give any oral or written statements, medical release, or have any other conversations with my employer, or the insurance carrier.

For me, the area of dispute was future medical care. I did not search out any other disability claims with social security or my personal insurance. I wanted to continue working in the nursing field. I loved nursing and I couldn't think of doing anything else. Besides, disability compensation was nowhere near my nurse's salary.

I was informed by the lawyer that the process was slow and I might not hear from him for many months. After a period of time, a hearing was scheduled for March 26, 2001. I don't recall much of that hearing except I answered a few questions and it lasted about twenty minutes. The attorneys did most of the work. I didn't hear anything again until December. In the meantime, my medical care was being covered. I continued to work on my master's degree and worked part time in the home health department.

In January 2002, a settlement was finally reached, and I was awarded future medical care plus a monetary award. I was totally surprised by the money. In June, I completed the master's degree requirements and I began employment at a community college as a nursing instructor. I entered the career path I thought would eliminate or at least reduce my exposure to latex. I was wrong.

Part II

Chapter 4

FROM RUBBER TREES TO LATEX GLOVES

The Rubber Story.

In Central America, as early as the 8th century, there is evidence of native Mayans using an elastic material. They made this substance by combining the milky liquid of native trees and vines, then added heat to create a solid, elastic mass. They found many uses for this new material. The Mayans would cut this material into thin strips and used them to wrap and carry bundles of sticks. They protected their feet by wrapping them with thick pieces of the pliable material. Female natives made jugs by smearing the sticky liquid over round clay forms. When the sticky substance dried the clay ball was smashed, leaving a water tight vessel. They also discovered that this material, when shaped into a ball, could bounce. There are remnants of ball fields in Chichén Itzá where they played their famous Mayan ball game using this new substance.

There are many versions of the game. One version written by Finney (2006) indicates the game was played to the death of the winner. The winning team's captain would offer his head to the losing team who would decapitate him. The Mayan's believed that this was a very honorable death and a quick route to heaven. Pieces of skull bones have been found near the ball fields.

Early European explorers were impressed with this substance but it wasn't until 1735 when Charles Marie de la Condamine, during his travels, recognized the importance of this sticky, milky white liquid. He was so astonished he sent specimens back to England.

English scientists discovered that this substance had many properties. The milky white colloid was named latex. It hardened when exposed to air, can be soft and sticky in warm weather, while brittle and stiff in cold weather. Over the next one hundred years, chemists tried to develop the liquid into a useful commodity. They experimented by adding different chemicals to the sticky substance. It is said that the Englishman, Joseph Priestly, named the substance "rubber" when he accidentally "rubbed out" some of his scientific pencil drawings with this material.

In 1823 Scottish born Charles Macintosh added a benzene chemical to the rubber solution and applied it to cloth, creating a waterproof fabric. This processed fabric still bears his name today, the "mackintosh". Many different clothing items were made with this coated fabric including shoes, life preservers, and canvas for backpacks and covers. However, the product still had a major fault: The Macintosh product would become stiff in cold weather and sticky in warm weather.

It was the vulcanization of rubber that made it a more useful commodity. The process was accidentally discovered by American Charles Goodyear in 1839. He was experimenting in his shop when he accidentally dropped raw rubber combined with white lead and sulfur on a hot stove. The result was a pliable product which could stretch and return to its original shape without being sticky or brittle. This was one of history's greatest accidental inventions. However, Goodyear had many financial problems and wasn't able to patent his product until January 30, 1844.

In the meantime, Thomas Hancock, another major English industrialist, established a rubber factory in England around 1820. He created the first rubber shredder or what is now called a "masticator" machine. The shredded rubber was used to make insulation. When he obtained a sample of Charles Goodyear's accidental invention, he replicated it and named the process "vulcanization" after Vulcan, the mythical Roman god of fire and smithery. He filed his patent in England on November 21, 1843 two months before Goodyear filed his in the USA. From then on the usefulness of rubber escalated.

Charles Goodyear never reaped financial benefit from his invention and he died in 1860 leaving his family in debt. He did not start the Goodyear Tire and Rubber Company. It was founded by Frank Seiberling, thirty-eight years after Charles Goodyear's death. Mr. Seiberling named the company in honor of Charles Goodyear.

Rubber can be obtained from many different tropical trees and plants. The best source is the *Hevea brasiliensis* tree. The largest source of this wild rubber tree is around the Amazon River in Central and South America.

Today, rubber is cultivated in large *Hevea brasiliensis* rubber tree plantations in Southeast Asia, Africa, India, South America and the Philippines. It is a billion dollar industry.

First Surgical Rubber Glove.

In the late 1890s a few rubber gloves were being made with vulcanized rubber but the gloves were heavy and ill fitting. These early gloves were used by utility workers and those working with chemicals. Some physicians used the gloves while performing autopsies to protect themselves from infectious disease. Surgeons tried using rubber gloves in surgery, but many felt the gloves were cumbersome and created more problems. They did not have the tactile feel and surgical wounds had to be made larger in order for the surgeon to manipulate the organs with gloves on. The gloves were not disposable and had to be washed and sterilized after each use. They had to be made in specific sizes: 6, 7, 8, etc. Universal acceptance and use of rubber gloves in surgery did not occur until the 1920s.

In the 1920s, the process of dipping items or forms in liquid rubber latex was discovered. One of the first products of this process was the balloon. The Tillotson Rubber Company in 1931 made the first "cat" balloon with ears and a painted face. These first balloons were used in parades and sold in toy stores. Tillotson made 5000 balloons in the first year in business. An especially important Tillotson product was coated cloth gloves and aprons.

Cloth gloves and aprons were "dipped" into liquid latex making the coated fabric an excellent barrier for the chemical or hazardous material worker. After the Second World War, Tillotson developed and manufactured the latex girdle, latex baby pants, and many other latex coated products by using the dipping method.

Disposable Latex Glove Manufacturing.

It wasn't until 1960 when the first disposable natural rubber latex (NRL) medical glove was developed by Tillotson Rubber Company. The advantage of this glove was that it was elastic and could stretch to fit most size hands. They could be made in generic sizes of small, medium, and large.

Smooth, clean ceramic formers or molds in the shape of fingers and hands are dipped in a tank full of latex sap mixed with chemicals. This process has several steps; dipping, drying, leaching, oven drying, wet powdering, and another tumbler drying phase. The length of time the formers are in the liquid latex tank determines the thickness of the glove.

After dipping, the coated formers are dried in an oven. This "vulcanizes" the latex. After the oven, the glove formers are dipped again in "leaching" water tanks. The water washes out the chemical residue and excess latex proteins. This important step differs with each glove manufacturer. The length of time and the use of fresh circulating water in the leaching bath affect the allergenicity of the glove. Longer leaching time reduces the allergens but can be costly for the manufacturer.

After the water bath, the gloves, still on the formers, are dried in ovens again. After drying, all gloves go through the wet-powder stage; they are covered with a wet cornstarch powder inside and out. The powder acts as a preservative for the glove, keeps the glove from sticking to itself, and makes the donning of the glove easier.

Next, they are removed from the molds and tumbled in heated dryers. The heat removes the excess powder and increases the elasticity of the gloves.

Powder-Free Latex Gloves.

Gloves labeled "powder-free" have the same initial steps but go through several additional water rinses. A chlorine bath rinse is added after the wet-powder stage to further reduce the powder and chemical residue. Then, the gloves are placed in the heated dryers again. They are removed from the formers, tested for defects, and packed in boxes by hand. Gloves are layered for easy removal from the boxes. A great web site explaining this process is http://www.medicalexamgloves.com /latex/manufacturing_process.html.

Allergenic Properties of Rubber.

The first documentation of rubber having allergenic properties was in an article written by Dr. John G. Downing published in the *New England Journal of Medicine* in 1933. He reported on surgeons getting dermatitis with itching and swelling of their hands after wearing surgical gloves. With further investigation, he found that several public utility linemen also manifested an itchy dermatitis and swollen hands after wearing rubber utility gloves. The linemen are required to wear rubber gloves when climbing utility poles. They wore short cotton gloves underneath the heavy rubber gloves. The rubber gloves were longer and extended over their wrist where the rubber came in direct contact with the skin. They all presented with the same type of reaction at their wrists; red, itchy skin with papules, raised pin-size solid lesions, vesicles, and fluid filled blisters. The glove manufacturers, when contacted, said they were aware of the problem. They have found that there was no specific causative factor. Each case reacted to different proteins in the gloves, and/or the chemicals used to vulcanize rubber. In some cases, the person even reacted to rubber vulcanized by the heat process. They had done considerable research on the problem and could not come up with a conclusion that was the same for all sensitive individuals.

In addition, each glove manufacturer uses different chemicals in the manufacturing process. It is difficult to determine which chemical is causing the allergic reactions. It has been found that the sensitive person can be allergic to the chemical and/or the latex proteins. Also, there are over 60 different latex proteins which make it difficult to determine the specific protein allergen. It is the leaching step that determines how allergenic the glove may be and it is this step that manufacturers shortened in order to meet the huge demand for gloves in the 1980s.

The differences in chemicals, leaching time, and the individual's sensitivity made it impossible to label a glove hypoallergenic, and the FDA in 1999 mandated the "hypoallergenic" label be removed from glove boxes.

Chapter 5

HISTORY OF RUBBER GLOVES IN HEALTH CARE

The history of cleanliness and sterile technique in healthcare is less than 150 years old. Prior to the middle nineteenth century, patient care—including surgeries—were performed with bare unwashed hands. Physicians wore their street clothes and perhaps used an apron.

Ignaz Semmelweis in 1846 was the first physician to promote hand washing. He identified that post-partum infection, called puerperal sepsis, was caused by unwashed hands and the transfer of infectious material from the physician's unwashed hands to the patient. He observed physicians and medical students performing surgeries and autopsies and then assisting with child birth without washing hands.

Before Louis Pasteur's germ theory was published in the 1850s, it was believed that infections were caused by spontaneous generation. After Pasteur identified microscopic bacteria in the air and on objects, and their relationship to causing fermentation, Joseph Lister in 1861 discovered the connection between fermentation and wound infections. He was the first to wash wounds and surgical instruments with carbolic acid.

He also recommended hand washing and the use of carbolic acid hand rinse before performing surgery. Surgical infection rates dropped almost in half.

In 1885 German-borne Heinrich Koch proved Pasteur's germ theory. He did this by linking a bacterium with a specific disease. All of this eventually, albeit slowly, changed healthcare practices.

Surgical Attire and Rubber Gloves.

In the1890s the first rubber surgical glove was manufactured. Ironically, the intention was to reduce the need for lengthy hand scrubbing with harsh soaps and the use of chemical washes before performing surgery; not for infection control.

A popular story regarding the first surgical glove use in the United States was from John Hopkins Hospital. A surgical nurse for a well known surgeon, William Halsted, had developed severe dermatitis from using harsh chemicals and soaps when scrubbing her hands before surgery. The surgeon asked Goodyear Rubber Company to make a pair of rubber surgical gloves. The gloves worked. Her dermatitis cleared. Eventually, other surgical technicians chose to wear gloves.

Not only did the surgical staff have less skin irritation, there was a noticeable drop in post-surgical infections and by 1894, John Hopkins became the first hospital in the United States to require all surgical staff to wear rubber gloves (Figure 3).

The natural rubber latex surgical glove was thick and bulky. The first *sterile* rubber glove was used around 1898 after Ernest von Bergmann discovered steam sterilization. The discovery of steam sterilization also allowed for sterile cloth gowns and masks to be used in surgery.

These early antiseptic techniques were not always accepted by all physicians. Many surgeons and hospitals were reluctant to change, even though Lister's hand washing techniques and the wearing of gloves continued to show a decline in infection rates.

Eventually, antiseptic technique changed to asepsis. Cleanliness slowly became the new paradigm in healthcare in the late nineteenth century. Florence Nightingale, the founder of modern nursing, during the 1860 Crimean War, proved that cleanliness of the patient's environment contributed significantly to the patient's recovery and the decrease in infection rates.

Still, sterile technique in surgery and the use of sterile gowns, gloves, and masks didn't become the norm until the 1920s. Physicians felt that wearing masks and gowns during surgery created a frightening atmosphere for the patient.

The flu pandemic of 1918 made physicians change their minds and use cloth masks for their own protection.

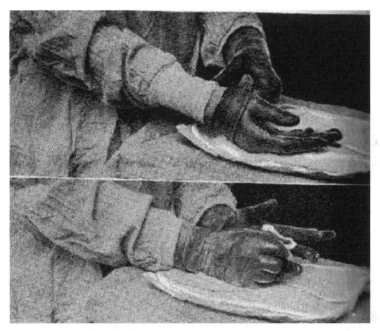

Figure 3. From *Eliason's Surgical Nursing* (p. 126), L.K. Ferguson and L.A. Sholtis, 1959, Philadelphia, PA: .JB Lippincott. Reprinted with permission.

Originally, surgical attire was white. The brightness of white was disturbing in the operating room, plus red blood against white was even more disturbing. In the 1950s the surgical gown color changed to green. This is when they became called "surgical greens" or "surgical scrubs." Despite this, street clothes were still worn under the cloth surgical gowns until the 1940s when the scrub uniform started to became the norm. Men wore green draw string pants and v-neck tops. The women wore cotton draw string dresses. Eventually, scrub pants and tops were available for women too.

Cleanliness and Asepsis.

By the 1960s hospitals were aseptic environments. There are two classifications of asepsis, medical and surgical. Medical asepsis means free of all *harmful* (pathogenic) bacteria while surgical asepsis or sterilization, means free of *all* bacteria—harmful, pathogenic, as well as non-harmful or non-pathogenic.

Cleanliness is the chief instrument of asepsis. This included cleanliness of the patient's total environment: room, bed linen, equipment, floors and walls. Personal cleanliness and hygiene of the hospital staff was also encouraged. Until the 1970s nurses and patient care staff wore white uniforms which are considered a symbol of cleanliness and professionalism. It was considered wrong to wear your uniform into public places.

Prior to the 1960s patient care items were washed, sterilized and reused; which was very labor intensive. Each individual hospital had large central supply departments where patient care items were cleaned and sterilized. Everything from glass syringes to bed pans was sterilized for reuse.

Chemical sterilization was used for items that could not withstand high temperatures and heat sterilization was used for items that would be affected by chemicals. The process for cleaning and sterilizing rubber gloves was time consuming and required additional equipment. For that reason, rubber gloves were only used in surgery and for sterile procedures. They were not used in providing routine daily patient care. Instead of using gloves while preparing a sterile field, long handled forceps were used to remove sterile items from their packages and placed on sterile fields. These large forceps were kept in metal containers of antiseptic solution. Only the tip of the forceps was considered sterile, therefore the handle of the forceps could be touched with bare hands. The solution in the container was changed daily (Figure 4). Rubber gloves were reused. After use, they were cleaned inside and out and washed by hand or in washing machines. After rinsing, they were dried either by hanging on a line or in large dryers. Gloves had to be turned inside out to dry both surfaces. When dry, they were powdered by hand or in a rotating drum machine (see Figure 5). Finally, they were checked for rips and pin holes and repaired with liquid latex. Then they were matched in size, wrapped appropriately in cloth muslin, and steam sterilized in autoclaves.

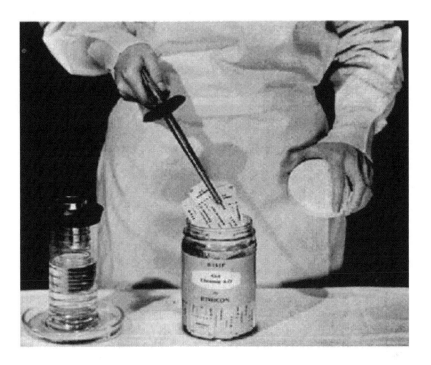

Figure 4. From *Eliason's Surgical Nursing* (p. 129), L.K. Ferguson and L.A. Sholtis, 1959, Philadelphia, PA: JB Lippincott. Reprinted with permission.

The biggest change in the delivery of healthcare came with the discovery of plastic and disposable patient care supplies. Single use items became the best design for infection control practices. Ironically, confining sick and infectious patients in a close environment, such as a hospital, increases the risk of. spreading infections to other patients. Hospital-acquired infections were costly to the hospital and to the patient and lengthened their stay. The biggest change in the delivery cost was always a concern. Disposable items were initially expensive, but the cleaning and sterilizing of reusable patient care items was labor and cost intensive.

Disposable Patient Care Items.

Disposable latex gloves became available in the 1960s; however, because of the cost, they still were not used for everyday patient care. Protective equipment such as gowns, mask and gloves were used only for known infectious patients who were isolated in separate hospital rooms. The primary concept of medical asepsis at this time was to prevent the spread of infection between patients. The fear of contracting a deadly disease was not a major concern for the hospital or staff. Hand washing was, and still is, the single most important method to prevent the spread of infection. In addition, procedures and techniques were taught and used by the staff to promote and maintain clean environments.

Blood-borne Pathogens Change Everything.

Changes in workplace aseptic practice again changed in the 1980s with the identification of blood-borne pathogens. Now the healthcare worker was at risk, and this risk could produce a significant consequence. The worker handling infected blood could acquire the infection if he had small cuts or lesion on his hands, or if he poked himself with a contaminated needle. Major changes were made in the handling of contaminated patient care items, needle and sharp disposal and, of course, the wearing of gloves.

At first it was difficult to remember to wear gloves. It was time consuming to find the gloves and stop to put them on and then again to stop and take them off when leaving the patient's room. In a busy healthcare setting this took extra seconds to complete. Non-sterile, powdered latex gloves were considered the best protection. Latex was considered the best barrier against chemicals and bacteria. Gloves became ubiquitous; on the medication carts, in the nurses station, and in the patient rooms. Nurses carried gloves in their pockets. Everyone from housekeeping staff to the physicians were constantly putting on and taking off latex gloves. In addition, the frequency of hand washing increased. Workers hands became red, irritated, and developed painful rashes.

The glove demand exploded. Glove usage went from thousands to billions per year. In order to meet the demand, manufacturers started to change steps in the manufacturing process. Shorter leaching and rinse time, and shorter shelf time left more latex proteins and chemicals in the gloves, increasing the allergenicity of the glove.

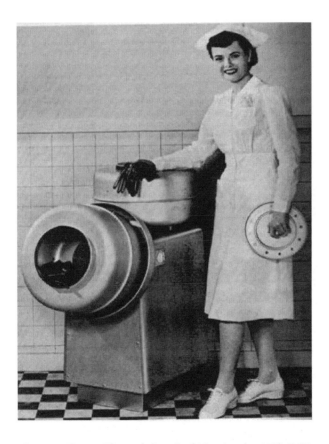

Figure 5. From *Eliason's Surgical Nursing* (p. 172), L.K. Ferguson and L.A. Sholtis, 1959, Philadelphia, PA: JB Lippincott. Reprinted with permission.

Part III

Chapter 6

THE ALLERGIC (HYPERSENSITIVITY) RESPONSE

Our amazing immune system quietly protects us against foreign substances, especially infectious diseases. It is a well tuned system which may break down and cause an inappropriate or an exaggerated hypersensitivity reaction to antigens, environmental, or from within us. Hypersensitivity is an altered immune response that results in disease or damage to the individual. Allergy, autoimmunity and alloimmunity are inappropriate reactions of the immune system. Allergy is a reaction to environmental antigens; autoimmunity is a reaction to self-antigens causing diseases such as lupus; and alloimmunity is an immune system response to blood transfusions, transplanted human tissue, or organs.

The immune system is complex and has many avenues of function. This author intends to try and simplify the immune system response specifically to the latex protein antigen. The reader is encouraged to refer to immunology textbooks if he or she feels the need for further explanation. For this chapter the author refers to two other references: *Understanding Pathophysiology* by Huether & McCance; and Dr R.F. Edlich's explanation of the allergic responses in his book *Medicine's Deadly Dust*.

There are four classifications of hypersensitivity. Type I is an IgE mediated response, also called Humoral Immune Response, Type II is a tissue specific response; Type III an immune complex mediated response and Type IV a cell mediated response. The latex allergic individual may have a Type I or Type IV allergic hypersensitivity. These are true allergic reactions. This discussion will be limited to these two types. The initial exposure to any antigen the body recognizes as a foreign substance causes a primary immune system response *with no* symptoms or visible reactions. If the exposure continues then the secondary and subsequent immune system response occurs *with* symptoms. The response can be immediate or delayed and may be interrelated. Delayed reactions can take several hours to appear.

Methods of exposure to latex proteins are: skin contact, gastrointestinal tract (eating), mucosal contact, such as frequent, invasive use of rubber catheters or condoms, and respiratory contact—inhalation of airborne latex particles.

Irritant Contact Dermatitis.

The frequent wearing of latex gloves combined with frequent hand washing may cause a local irritant contact dermatitis, which, is not in itself, considered an allergy but which may be an avenue to acquiring a true allergic hypersensitivity. If this phase is recognized and no further contact is made with latex, an allergy can be avoided.

This irritation is caused by powder lubricants used in latex gloves and frequent hand washing. It is manifested by red, dry, itchy hands. Often there are skin cracks, rashes and open lesions. The reaction is limited to the area of contact. Hand dermatitis is the most frequent initial complaint of latex glove wearers. If exposure continues, the non-intact skin allows latex proteins to enter the body system and cause either a cell mediated Type IV response, an IgE, Type I mediated response, or both.

Cell Mediated Hypersensitivity Type IV.

The immune system's main player in this type of reaction is the T-Lymphocyte cells, not antibodies. T-Cells are white blood cells that "attach and destroy." This reaction occurs in response to cancer tumor cells, metals, or chemical antigens. Small molecular weight antigens, in this case, latex proteins, are called haptens. They are too small to create an allergic response by themselves. Once in contact with the skin, they combine with larger skin protein cells called Langerhan cells. This combined cell becomes immunogenic. These cells degrade the latex protein and float into the lymph system where they meet up with T-lymphocytic cells, or T-cells. The degraded protein product attaches to a T-cell. The T-cell thus becomes sensitized and migrates back to the skin. There is no visible reaction at this time. The T-cell is sensitized (loaded) and waiting for another latex antigen to pull the trigger. With another exposure, the antigen binds to the skin protein cell, which carries the latex protein to the sensitized T-cell. This trigger phase causes the sensitized T-cell to manufacture chemicals such as cytokines. These cytotoxic chemicals set off an inflammatory cascade response and stimulate the phagocytic (killer) cells, macrophages, which may attach tumor cells and cause destruction of tissue. This phagocytic and inflammatory response is responsible for skin tissue damage. Thus, Type IV is an Allergic Contact Dermatitis. Interestingly, this process led to the discovery of the Tuberculosis skin test. The delayed inflammatory response indicates a positive reaction to the TB antigen used in skin testing. This means the person is sensitized to TB and in need of further diagnostic tests.

The most common and well known environmental Type IV allergen is poison ivy. The poison ivy plant proteins react with normal skin proteins and start a cell-mediated response as described above, resulting in a destruction of tissue and causing dermatitis in the area of contact. Other Type IV environmental allergens are certain metals and chemicals. In the case of latex gloves, the chemicals used in manufacturing can be the cause of Type IV reactions (See Figure 6).

Each latex glove manufacturer, as discussed previously, may use many different chemicals and have variable leaching times. This is why someone may react to one manufacturer's glove and not another. The length of time the glove spends in the leaching line determines how much of the chemical and latex proteins will be washed out from the glove. Several wash cycles are needed to wash out the latex proteins and chemicals adequately.

Type IV reactions consist of severe dermatitis and itching at the area of contact. There may be some fluid filled vesicles and oozing of clear fluid. The induced inflammatory response increases blood flow resulting in swelling and erythema. The response may be delayed two to four hours. This time may shorten with each repeated exposure. The dermatitis could spread to adjacent areas and persist for weeks without continued or repeated exposure.

Type IV Cell Mediated Response

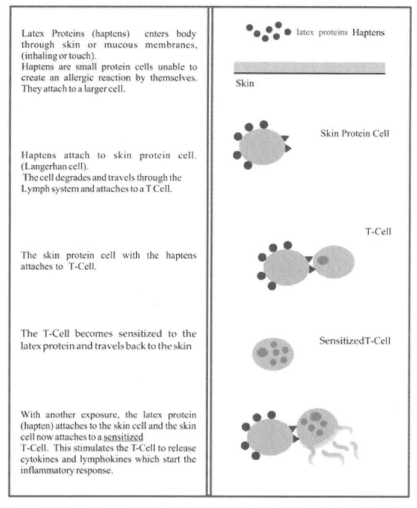

Latex Proteins (haptens) enters body through skin or mucous membranes, (inhaling or touch). Haptens are small protein cells unable to create an allergic reaction by themselves. They attach to a larger cell.

Haptens attach to skin protein cell. (Langerhan cell). The cell degrades and travels through the Lymph system and attaches to a T Cell.

The skin protein cell with the haptens attaches to T-Cell.

The T-Cell becomes sensitized to the latex protein and travels back to the skin

With another exposure, the latex protein (hapten) attaches to the skin cell and the skin cell now attaches to a sensitized T-Cell. This stimulates the T-Cell to release cytokines and lymphokines which start the inflammatory response.

latex proteins Haptens

Skin

Skin Protein Cell

T-Cell

Sensitized T-Cell

Figure 6. Adapted from Edlich, R.F. (1997), *Medicine's Deadly Dust*; Heuther, S.E. & McCance, K.L. (2008), *Understanding Pathophysiology*. Copyright 2012, Margaret Konieczny.

IgE mediated Hypersensitivity Type I.

IgE antibody, B Lymphocytic cells, mast cells, and histamine are the main players in this immune system overreaction. True allergy is manifested by the production of IgE antibodies. They are specific to a certain allergen. It is the most common and most serious life threatening reaction. IgE is an antibody that protects against large parasites and is also produced against environmental antigens. IgE and mast cell products mediate the Type I response. The main purpose of IgE is to cause an inflammatory response.

When the specific environmental antigen exposure occurs, the latex protein (hapten) attaches to the skin protein cell, Langerhan Cell. This antigen cell attaches to T-Cells and B-lymphocytic cells. B-Cells change to plasma cells. These cells are now sensitized. The plasma cell produces IgE antibodies specific to the causative antigen. The allergic individual may have many different specific IgE antibodies floating in their immune systems. The free floating IgE quickly binds to the mast cell receptor sites. Once a large amount of IgE antibodies are attached to the mast cell, the cell is considered sensitized. This phase may last for years and has no symptoms. Mast cells carry several chemicals, one of which is histamine.

When a subsequent exposure occurs, the antigen attaches directly to IgE molecules sitting on a mast cell instead of the sensitized B-Cell. When the antigen cell attaches to two IgE molecules, it causes a bridging effect which alters the mast cells membrane. This bridging effect causes the mast cell membrane to break down, degranulate, and release histamine and other chemicals into the blood stream (see Figure 7). These highly reactive chemicals are responsible for the *systemic*, anaphylactic allergic reactions. Areas of the body that have the most mast cells have the most reactions. They are the respiratory tract, skin, and gastrointestinal tract (See Figure 7).

Histamine causes systemic dilatation of the blood vessels. When the blood vessels dilate, fluid and blood cells leak out into the tissues causing swelling and inflammation. The dilatation of the blood vessels in the respiratory system causes pharyngeal swelling, swelling of the lung mucosa, bronchial swelling, and increased secretions. This process decreases and constricts the size of the bronchial airways. The symptoms of bronchial constriction are wheezing and shortness of breath, with a feeling of suffocation. Reactions can progress to anaphylaxis; respiratory distress, throat closure, hypotension, and possibly death if not treated immediately.

The skin reactions include, dermatitis, itching, inflammation—with sense of skin irritability, burning and stinging, plus angioedema (swelling of the face or total body). Included are eye symptoms of conjunctivitis, itchy, watery eyes, peri-orbital swelling with erythema and rhinitis. Gastrointestinal symptoms of nausea, vomiting, cramps and diarrhea may also occur. The reaction may occur immediately after exposure or can be delayed one to two hours. Individuals who are genetically predisposed to allergies are called *atopic*. These individuals have higher quantities of IgE and more receptors on their mast cells. Their airway and skin are more responsive to antigen stimuli. This is the theory why atopic individuals are more apt to have serious reactions to latex proteins.

Cross-Reactivity/Fruit Syndrome.

Latex allergic individuals probably will have an IgE mediated response to certain foods that have the same or similar antigen structure. Our immune system recognizes the food proteins as a latex allergen and will illicit the same type of response as a Type I hypersensitivity, and will have the same reactive skin, respiratory, or gastrointestinal symptoms mentioned in the previous chapter.

It has been discovered that protein allergens are associated with the defense enzymes a plant will produce. If a plant or tree is injured, the plant produces an enzyme that protects the plant from further injury by microbes or fungi. In the harvesting of natural rubber latex from the *Hevea brasiliensis* tree, the bark of the tree is "wounded" causing the tree to produce defensive enzymes. These enzymes are harvested with the milky latex fluid. It has been found that seven of the thirteen latex allergen proteins are defensive proteins. This defensive enzyme has properties that are similar to many plants including common foods. These protective enzymes are potent allergens. Many tropical fruits and vegetables have similar defensive enzymes.

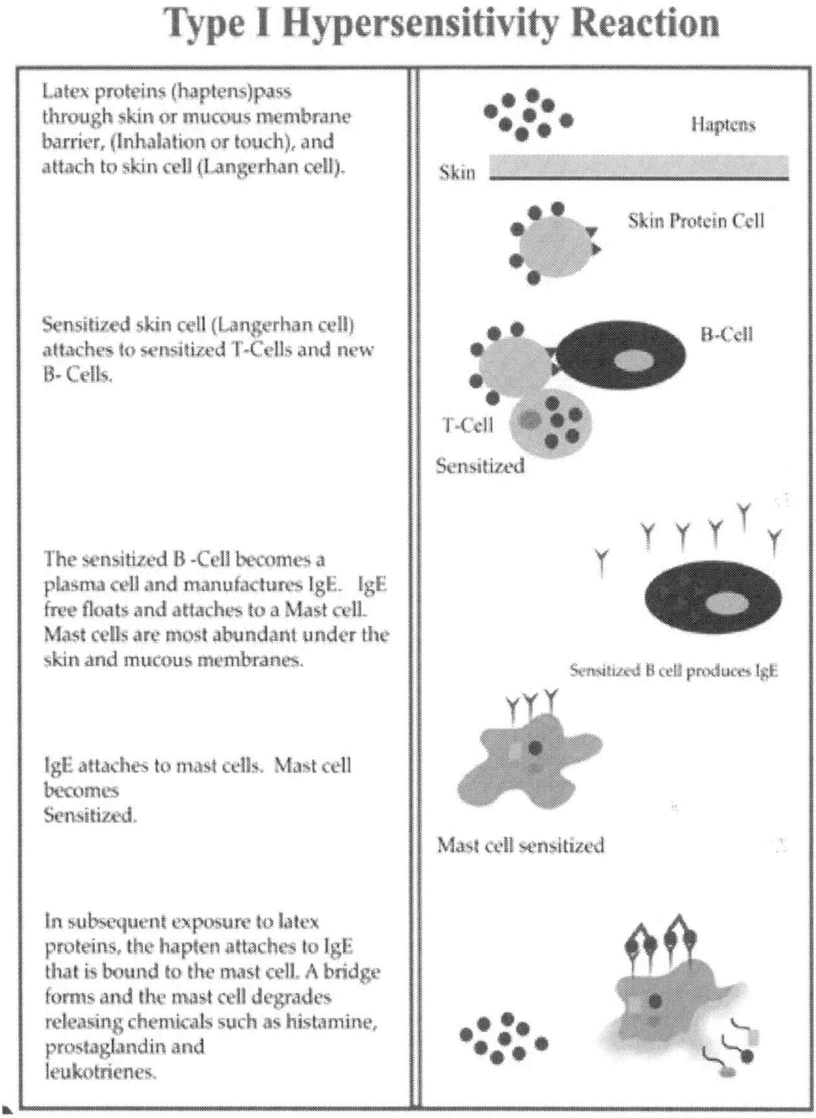

Type I Hypersensitivity Reaction

Latex proteins (haptens) pass through skin or mucous membrane barrier, (Inhalation or touch), and attach to skin cell (Langerhan cell).

Haptens

Skin

Skin Protein Cell

Sensitized skin cell (Langerhan cell) attaches to sensitized T-Cells and new B- Cells.

B-Cell

T-Cell

Sensitized

The sensitized B -Cell becomes a plasma cell and manufactures IgE. IgE free floats and attaches to a Mast cell. Mast cells are most abundant under the skin and mucous membranes.

Sensitized B cell produces IgE

IgE attaches to mast cells. Mast cell becomes Sensitized.

Mast cell sensitized

In subsequent exposure to latex proteins, the hapten attaches to IgE that is bound to the mast cell. A bridge forms and the mast cell degrades releasing chemicals such as histamine, prostaglandin and leukotrienes.

Figure 7. Adapted from Edlich, R.F. (1997), *Medicine's DeadlyDust*;Heuther,S.E. &McCance,K.L.(2008),*Understanding Pathophysiology*. Copyright 2012, Margaret Konieczny.

This association is called cross-reactive syndrome or fruit-syndrome. One may be allergic to several of the foods and may not have any allergic reactions to others on the list. One may have a severe reaction to one, and a mild reaction to another. It is important to note that if you are latex sensitive you must be aware that you might have a reaction to some of the cross reactive foods. Conversely, if you have an allergy to any of these foods you might develop an allergy to latex or you may have a latex sensitivity and don't know it. The chart below lists which of the foods are of high, moderate, or low probability (Figure 8).

CROSS-REACTIVE FOODS

HIGH	**MODERATE**	**LOW**
BANANAS	MELONS	PEAR
AVOCADOS	TOMATOES	PEACH
KIWI	APPLE	CHERRY
CHESTNUTS	CARROTS	STRAWBERRY
	PAPAYA	MANGO
	CELERY	APRICOTS
	POTATO	GRAPES
		PAPAYA

**Figure 8. For more information visit w.latexallergyresources.org.
Copyright 2012, Margaret Konieczny.**

PART IV

Chapter 7

MY LIFE 2002-2009

2002-2009.

In the fall of 2002 I left home health and began teaching nursing students at a local community college. I was doing well and wanted to move on with my life. I continued to be vigilant and modified my life for any known latex exposure. I informed my new employer of my latex allergy. In the meantime, I discovered the school's nursing lab had supplies that contained latex rubber, including latex gloves both powdered and non-powdered. I asked the school to replace the gloves and supplies. Over the years, the supplies were slowly exchanged. There were times when the school would receive free donated patient care supplies, and many latex products were included. I was constantly on alert for these items. When I discussed this with the program's director I felt I was getting a skeptical response. I knew I had to be personally responsible in avoiding exposure. I also came to realize that the general public still thinks that a latex allergy consists only of hand dermatitis. If they haven't seen severe reactions,, they just don't know. This realization made me reflect on how I respond to people who tell me they have an allergy. I realized I too could be skeptical and I found someone else's allergy very inconvenient, especially if I had to alter my actions to accommodate them. It is annoying. So, I understood everyone else's skepticism of my allergy. Allergies are problematic for the sufferer and those around them.

After a while, I forgot how severe my reactions could be. I took pictures of myself starting back in 1998, and I am glad I did. I look at them from time to time to remind myself of the reactions. In retrospect, I should have posted my pictures on the walls of the nursing lab so others could see and would understand, but I didn't make a big deal of it because I wanted to leave it in my past and move on. Health care facilities were becoming latex-safe. I felt if I avoided latex in my own personal space, I would be fine. I had a few more years to work until I retired and I wanted to teach nursing and end my career doing what I loved.

Over the next few years my reactions were small and manageable. In addition, the time I spent in the lab and clinical sites was less than half of the semester so, when a reaction occurred, I had time to recover. I treated myself following Dr. Saylor's prescribed drug regime and with over the counter cortisone creams and eye drops. Occasionally I would feel short of breath and would use a rescue inhaler. It never significantly impacted my daily activity. Things continued in this manner for the next four years.

2007.

In 2007 the reactions were becoming more bothersome. I had longer periods of reactivity and an increase in asthma symptoms. I soon learned that with continued exposure to latex, sensitivity increases and the allergic response is more severe. I had not seen my allergist since 2003 and my medications were outdated. I made an appointment to see Dr. Saylor on June 14, 2007. I told him I had multiple small reactions in the past but they were manageable. Some of those reactions were while in clinical sites and some were in other areas of my life. One of those exposures was during an outpatient procedure using EKG monitoring pads. I had skin reactions in the area of pad placement. When I called the procedure nurse to report the reaction, she informed me that the pads were not labeled latex-free. Usually products that are latex free are labeled "Latex free".

I also told Dr. Saylor of two more cross-reactive foods I identified through trial and error. I cannot eat avocados and kiwi. He renewed my medications and again advised me to be more vigilant. I was to see him again in one year. All was well again until the fall of 2008.

2008.

In the fall of 2008 I was supervising students in an extended care facility. That year they had powder-free latex gloves as well as nitrile gloves available for patient care. The staff and students used both the latex and non-latex gloves. I avoided latex as best as I could; however, I was working with others who were wearing them and I was touching the objects they touched. By the end of the eight week rotation my face became crimson again with a burning, stinging, rash, and itchy, puffy, watery eyes. In addition I felt short of breath. I treated myself as I always did; knowing the semester would be over soon and I would recover.

I did not get better. Over the Christmas holiday, I acquired a respiratory infection and had to use my inhaler often. I suspected the use of latex gloves in the extended care facility might have compromised my asthma and the respiratory infection added to the injury. I couldn't say for sure.

I also looked at what was happening in my personal life. Latex products are ubiquitous. I may have come in contact with something I didn't recognize as latex. Later, I realized, I handled carpet padding in my home which was made of natural rubber latex.

This was the beginning of a super sensitive period for me. I tried to ignore it, deny it, and look for other reasons for my reaction. I kept believing the reactions would stop. They did not.

2009-10.

In January 2009, I continued to feel short of breath. My eyes watered and the facial redness, swelling and itching continued. I spent some time at my daughter's house helping her with her new infant. I was trying to ignore how I felt. I was hoping resolution would come soon.

My daughter's house had many steps and she lives at sea level. I kept blaming my shortness of breath on the stairs and the difference in altitude. I had paroxysmal atrial fibrillation and I thought that might contribute to the shortness of breath. However, upon reflection, the periods of the arrhythmia did not correlate with the periods of shortness of breath.

I kept looking for other reasons for this continued reaction. I looked at items in her home that might have latex content: items such as baby bottles and nipples and pacifiers. I could not identify any one specific item. It was a difficult time as I couldn't say for sure I had a latex exposure. I was feeling depressed as I didn't recover from the last school semester as I had hoped.

The winter semester started in the middle of January. For the first two weeks of the semester I taught students in the school's nursing lab. Then clinical practice started the last week of January. I continued to feel short of breath and I tried to ignore it. I could not get this reaction under control. By February, I noticed I was purse lip breathing while doing house work. With no relief, and with despondent resolve, I made an appointment to see Dr. Saylor on February 17, 2009.

When I saw him my rash was severe. It was diffuse all over my body, shoulders, neck, face, legs and waist. I told him I was short of breath since December and recently I started wheezing. He performed a modified PFT test and I failed it miserably. His response scared me and I told him so. He said I scared him! He would not let me drive home until I took the first dose of prednisone. In addition to the rescue inhaler, albuterol, he prescribed a cortisone inhaler.

I was perplexed as to why my allergic reaction was persisting. I reviewed my life again and the only exposure I could positively identify was the use of latex gloves by the students and staff at the extended care facility back in December. Currently, I was supervising students at the acute care facility which deemed itself to be latex-safe. So, I went back to work. While at the hospital on the next week, I went to get a pair of sterile gloves in order to assist a student with a sterile procedure.

I stopped in my tracks. The package label stated *sterile latex* gloves. Among them were packages labeled *powdered latex gloves*. I was astonished. I could not help the student.

When I asked the nursing managers about this they said the physicians requested latex gloves. That was it. I found the reason why my symptoms continued and intensified. I was being exposed to aerosolized latex from the use of powdered latex gloves in the hospital.

On February 24, 2009, my next visit to Dr. Saylor, I told him of my discovery. He restated that I could not work in any space that was not latex-safe and he wrote a note to that effect to my employer. I was devastated. I was fearful of losing my job. I hoped that I could finish my career without any further latex exposure problems.

Employment Issues Revisited.

The school accommodated me and took me out of clinical rotations. I only worked in the nursing lab and continued to teach in the classroom. My symptoms continued. I was on and off prednisone for the next two months. Now all latex items were suspect, whether I used them personally or not. I discovered latex gloves again in the school's lab and had them removed. I was teaching students in the lab using our high tech manikins. These manikins "breathe" with rubber, balloon-like lungs; the balloons expand and the chest rises. A power-driven box creates the lung sounds. The student can hear lung sounds with each "inspiration and expiration." They are taught to identify different lung sounds. I had worked with these manikins in January. Now, in March, while using these manikins, my face again became very red, swollen and itchy. I contacted the manikin manufacturer's representative; he indicated the rubber lungs did not "breathe." However, he did agree that the manikins have bellows which expand the balloon-like lungs, and makes the chest rise. With this discovery, I was relieved of the lab assignment and restricted to my office. In spite of this, I could not get the reaction under control even with bouts of prednisone therapy.

In May, I had a meeting with the college administrators. I had been asking for this meeting since March. Each time I wanted to discuss my future with the nursing program director, she kept referring me to the human resource department. She was very non-committal. I was feeling frustrated that we couldn't work out a plan for the next year. A few emails went back and forth between me and the HR director, discussing my latex allergy.

Finally, I insisted on a meeting to determine my future at the college. When the meeting was set up, I thought it would be between me and the HR director and possibly my nursing director. When I arrived at the meeting, to my surprise, the room was full. In addition to HR and the nursing director, the vice-president of the college and the dean of instruction were in attendance. Apparently, I wasn't grasping the enormity of my situation. After the meeting, I told the HR Director I was angry that he hadn't informed me who would be in attendance.

Despite my feelings of intimidation, I remained calm and presented my request. I wanted to work another two years before retirement. I approached the group about changing my position to the college's "phased-in retirement program." The program allows a faculty member, nearing retirement, to work sixty to eighty percent of their current work load and receive full time benefits. They could do this for two years only and then retire. I told them I could teach classroom nursing theory and teach in labs that were held in classrooms or clinics which were latex-safe. The nursing director told me she would not alter the schedules of the other nursing faculty to accommodate me. So there it was. The reality of her position finally surfaced. The vice-president said the only other way was for me to resign and apply for an adjunct teaching position (which would be at a lower salary.); however, there aren't any adjunct positions in the nursing program and I did not qualify to teach anything else. I was tenured. Didn't that mean anything? This confirmed my suspicions. I knew I wasn't the favorite nursing professor as I had disagreed with the nursing director on many occasions. The limitations my allergy required seemed to be a good out for her.

Since I didn't resign, I was placed on sick leave for two weeks which would last until the end of the semester. I was sent by the human resource director to their Occupational Health Physician. He told me and the school that I was to avoid latex at all cost. The school then placed me on an earned, extended, medical leave until February 2010. It was suggested by the human resource director that I contact the school's disability insurance. I did, and was denied benefits. The disability insurance company told me that since I could work in another capacity, such as consulting, I did not qualify for disability benefits. As long as there was a *possibility* I could work, they would not give me any benefits.

I felt deflated and in a Catch-22: I had a disability and couldn't work in latex environments but could work in other areas of nursing. Who would hire a latex allergic nurse in any capacity?

Chapter 8

WORKERS' COMPENSATION REVISITED

I did not file for Workers' Compensation with this employer as I had an open case with the California Workers' Compensation Insurance Company. In reality, I couldn't blame the college for my allergy; I just wanted them to accommodate my disability. I did contact a Nevada Workers' Compensation Lawyer to discuss my options. She told me I missed the filing period for Workers' Compensation, so I couldn't file if I wanted to. She also told me Nevada is a "right to work state" and my employer could terminate me even if I was tenured. She suggested I look at the school's policy for tenured faculty. I could tell she wasn't too interested in getting involved.

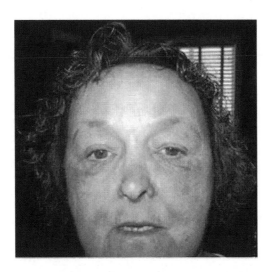

Figure 9. Post hair salon visit / hair coloring.
Copyright 2012, Margaret Konieczny.

The rest of 2009 was not good. Over the next few months, I had reactions to things I hadn't reacted to in the past. I had a reaction when I had my hair dyed (See Figure 9). When trying to understand why, I discovered a chemical, phenylenediamine, used in hair dye, is also used as a chemical accelerator in the manufacturing of late rubber gloves.

In July of that year I wore a new summer top with Lycra fibers and had a severe contact dermatitis reaction. After some research, I found Lycra is Spandex and "cases of dermatitis, due to Lycra/Spandex, have been traced to rubber or rubber processing chemicals added in the manufacturing of the synthetic fiber" (Groce, 1996). When I reacted to the Spandex bathing suit in 1998, I thought Spandex and latex was the same. Not so. Apparently, it is the chemicals I was reacting to; a Type IV reaction. These chemicals were identified during the skin testing I had done back in 1998; however, because of the lack of information about latex allergy, no relationship was made.

One month later in August 2009, a major reaction occurred while I was at my nursing school reunion in South Bend, Indiana. The first day in South Bend, I met with several old grade school classmates for lunch in a local restaurant. I had not seen some of these ladies for forty years and it seemed like it was just five years ago. We had lunch and sat in the restaurant for three hours and talked. Later that evening at the reunion, my face became scarlet red. By 10 p.m. my face and eyes began to swell. By morning, I had a round basketball face. The burning and throbbing was intense. The skin blistered and began to weep a clear fluid. My eyes were almost swollen shut. I tried all night to control the reaction by using cool compresses on my face. I used hydrocortisone cream and I took my miracle pill, Vistaril. Nothing helped. At this time I did not carry any prednisone tablets or an EpiPen® (Figure 10.1, 10.2).

I was devastated. *"Not again!"* I said. I looked awful and felt worse. At six a.m., I drove myself to the hospital. The ER nurses took one look at me and I was admitted. I told them of my latex allergy history. They were understanding and sympathetic. The doctor was not. He thought it was poison ivy. I was shocked. I recounted all the things I had done prior my admittance to the ER. I was not out walking in any fields. The reaction seemed to start shortly after I left the restaurant. By late evening my face

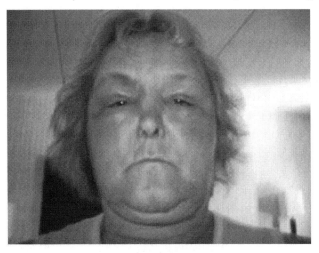

Figure 10.1 Post-restaurant visit.
fiCopyright 2012, Margaret Konieczny.

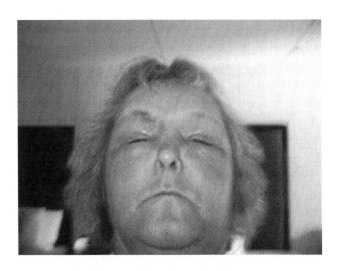

Figure 10.2. Post-restaurant visit.
Copyright 2012, Margaret Konieczny.

was red and began to sting and burn. I reviewed everything thing I did that day. I even checked the bedding and pillows at the hotel. They did not have any latex material. (Latex foam mattresses and pillows can still be used at hotels.) I retraced my steps, and the only place I could not rule out was the restaurant.

Since I could not say for sure how I got the latex exposure, the ER doctor kept thinking it was a poison ivy reaction. I was upset that he kept referring to poison ivy. I did not know at the time, Type IV latex allergic hypersensitivity reactions look like poison ivy reactions. I don't think the doctor realized this either, as he did not make the connection. The skin, in the area of contact with poison ivy, is usually swollen, itchy, and red, with weepy blisters. With my reaction, he must have thought I had my face in it!

The ER doctor diagnosed it as "Delayed Hypersensitivity Reaction" and did not mention any causative exposure. He prescribed prednisone and told me to follow up with my allergist when I got home. Luckily, I did not have any respiratory symptoms.

After my trip to the ER, I called the restaurant and spoke with the hostess. I told her a half truth. I told her I had a latex allergy and wanted to eat at the restaurant. Before I could, I needed to know if they used latex gloves. I didn't want to tell her I already had a reaction after eating there. I was afraid she wouldn't talk to me. She was very helpful and told me they did use gloves in the kitchen area. She read the label on a box of gloves and confirmed they were latex. As we talked, I mentioned powdered gloves were the worst for latex allergy sufferers. She then said, *"Oh, the box says they are slightly powdered."* *"Oh my God,"* I said to myself. *"This is it. This is the cause of my reaction."* In a way, I was relieved to know the cause. I explained how serious the reactions can be and how important it was not to use latex gloves in her restaurant. She said she would talk to the owners about using different gloves in the future.

I did not attend the rest of the reunion activities. I stayed in the hotel for the rest of the day. When the swelling went down the next day, I met with some old nursing friends, called family members, and made isolated trips in the city until I was to fly home two days later.

I followed up with my allergist, continued a prescribed prednisone regime, and began to heal. Now I avoid eating out. I call restaurants before I go. Surprisingly, about a third of the restaurants I called use latex gloves. If I am meeting friends for lunch, I tell them I need a restaurant that doesn't use latex gloves. My friends have been accommodating, even though it is an inconvenience for them.

Over the next few months my symptoms never fully went away. There was a persistent low grade effect. My eyes continued to be watery and itchy. The skin around my eyes remained crimson and puffy. I continued to look for any hidden latex in the products I used. I discovered my golf club grips are made from rubber. I replaced the rubber grips with synthetic.

That December, I had surgery for atrial fibrillation and informed the hospital of my allergy and gave them a picture for my chart. They were extremely accommodating; all the surgical staff, doctors, and floor nurses. I survived that hospitalization without any consequences, until I went home to my son's house and ate a fruit salad that included mangos. Mangos are on the list of cross reactive foods and I have been avoiding them. I did not realize they were in the fruit salad until it was too late. Two hours later, I had a reaction. I cannot tell you how disturbing that was. I was just home from the hospital after major surgery with no problems, and then in my son's home, I have a reaction. How crazy!

The reactions kept coming and grew in severity. From December 2009 till May of 2010, I continued to have major reactions about every month to 6 weeks. As one reaction healed another began. The skin reaction would start slowly and would peak by the third day. Disturbingly, the rash and itchy, puffy eyes would last weeks. I spent many nights awake with intense burning, stinging, and itching of the skin on my face and neck. I felt like my body was out of control. The skin felt uneasy and seemed to have a heightened sensitivity. I became super sensitive to any level of latex in the environment.

And the reactions continued. I reacted to prepackaged foods handled by workers using latex gloves at the processing plant. I reacted to tomatoes packaged by a certain tomato farm. When I looked up their website they had pictures of their workers wearing what appeared to be latex gloves (Latex gloves are manufactured in one color, a light tan.). There were other times when I just couldn't identify the causative agent.

In March of 2010, I was cutting back a ground cover plant in my back yard. It is called periwinkle. I love this plant-it is pretty in the spring, green all winter, and very hardy. It survives almost any kind of abuse. I have touched this plant many times before. This time I was using gloves, and at other times I just used my bare hands. I had a cold and I was touching my face frequently to wipe my nose. Two hours later, I could feel my face become hot, sting, burn and then literally "pop" out with a rash and swelling. It was a slow but progressive response. In addition, I became short of breath. It reminded me of Bruce Banner who had visual body changes as he "popped" into the green Incredible Hulk.

Again I reviewed the last couple of hours to determine the causative agent. Could it be that plant? It was the only new thing I did that day. I researched the internet for information on periwinkle. Again, I had another revelation. The web site stated, "Periwinkle is a plant in the Apocynaceae family. Many of these plants are found in tropical and temperate regions. The sap of these plants is milky white latex, which is used for medicinal purposes and for manufacturing rubber. The sap is often toxic" (http://theseedsite.co.uk/ apocy naceae.html), and here it is in my own back yard! I was amazed and now worried about how sensitive I had become and what I would find next (Figure 11).

I made several trips to Dr. Saylor that spring. I was placed on prednisone but as soon as I stopped the prednisone the reactions would start again. My asthma became severe and I was using my rescue inhaler daily. He strongly suggested Xolair injections, a very expensive IgE binding drug used for IgE allergic asthma. This drug is "off label" and not FDA approved. Xolair binds free IgE before it attaches to the mast cell preventing the mast cell from releasing histamine (see chapter six.) In spite of the possible side effect of anaphylaxis, Dr. Saylor felt it was my best chance for recovery. I was hesitant because it must be administered every two weeks at a physician's office, clinic, or hospital infusion center. For me, that meant traveling 200 miles round trip to Sacramento. In addition, at the time, Workers'

Compensation denied my medical benefits and we were in litigation again. The injections would cost around $5000.00 each. Fortunately, I had recently become eligible for Medicare. They would pay for the injections

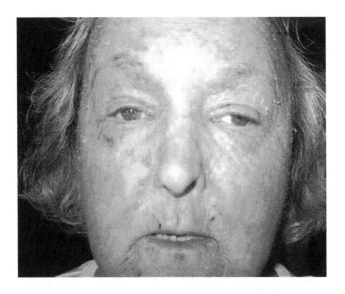

Figure 11. Post-gardening.
Copyright 2012, Margaret Konieczny.

and my supplemental insurance would cover the balance. This was good news as I was miserable and needed to start the injections. I knew I couldn't stay on prednisone forever and I couldn't wait for Workers' Compensation to start paying for the drug. The reactions were becoming my worse nightmare. I agreed to the treatment and started the Xolair injections on May 1st, 2010.

In addition, back in February 2010, when my medical leave expired, I was terminated from my teaching position because I could not complete the job description as written and the college would not accommodate me. They indicated their nursing faculty job description includes teaching in the classroom, laboratory, and clinical sites. Since I could not teach in clinical sites, I could not perform the "essential functions" of the job. They would not change other faculty's schedules to accommodate me.

In March of 2010, Workers' Compensation insisted that my exposures were non-industrial and they would not cover the medical cost for treatment. My original law firm was contacted by the Workers' Compensation insurance carrier and another round of legal conversations began. I went through depositions, QME (Qualified Medical Examiner) evaluations, hearings and lots of waiting. We argued that the original injury was work related and it is "permanent and stationary" meaning I have a permanent disability. I would be affected by latex in any environment for the rest of my life. Besides, the original settlement was for future medical care and did not stipulate only while employed at the original employer.

In this legal round, I was evaluated by a QME who was certified and worked for the State of California, Department of Industrial Relations, and Division of Occupational Medicine. The Workers' Compensation Insurance carrier chose this doctor for me.

This stuffy-seeming doctor, who reminded me of Ichabod Crane, acknowledged that I had a latex allergy, but he created doubt on whether my current symptoms—especially asthma—were related to the original industrial injury. Because of his report Workers' Compensation denied my claim. It took him four months to complete his report and in the meantime my private insurance and Medicare paid my bills.

I was entitled to another opinion by a physician of my choice. I found another independent QME. He is a well-recognized professor of medicine in the Department of Allergy and Immunology, Division of Occupational Health Services at the University of San Francisco. I was examined by this physician on June 28, 2010. He stated *"but for Ms Konieczny's latex allergy injury of 1997, she would not require treatment for her current symptoms due to respiratory and skin problems."* In addition, he stated, *"absent her allergy (latex) she would not need ongoing treatment with prednisone, inhaled bronchodilators and Xolair injections."* The argument was finally settled that fall. Workers' Compensation finally agreed to authorize my medical care.

During the first two months of treatment I was still on low dose prednisone. I was doing OK. My asthma was under control, but my facial rash and redness persisted. I had noticed the nurses at the infusion center used non-powdered latex gloves when working with chemotherapy drugs, and used non-latex, nitrile gloves when caring for me. The nurses considered this a latex-safe environment.

I was in a dilemma. I needed the injections, and there wasn't anywhere else to go. I did not want to stay in the department too long. The protocol for Xolair injections states that the patient has to remain in the controlled environment for one hour post injection to observe for any anaphylaxis. I cut that down to thirty to forty-five minutes.

Then one particular day they were very busy and I noticed the latex glove use was up. In addition, I noticed the housekeeping staff was using these gloves when cleaning the patient care units. That day, I was in the department about two hours. That evening my faced broke out again and the burning itching returned although somewhat muted. I notified Dr. Saylor. When was I going to learn that *any* latex in close proximity to me is not good for me? I need to be proactive for myself. Research shows that an individual with a Type I allergy to latex can just walk into a room where latex is being used and have a reaction. I don't have to touch it.

Before Dr. Saylor could change the facility location he received an offer for a medical position in another city. A position he couldn't refuse so he quit his private practice. I had some anxiety over breaking the bond between him and me. He was my physician for 12 years. He took good care of me. I didn't want to change doctors. I didn't think I could find another allergist who would work with Workers' Compensation Insurance. But I was lucky. I found an allergist in my locale that was willing to accept my case. It was time to find a physician closer to home.

It was another three months before I could start the injections again. The transition took time. During the period off Xolair, I had low grade persistent reactions of itchy, watery, puffy eyes, dermatitis, and asthma.

While off Xolair, I had a routine eye exam by an optometrist; he noticed my allergic looking eyes. He was sympathetic and prescribed a cortisone eye ointment. I was to apply a minute amount of the eye ointment to just the outer lids and not in the eye, for ten days only. It is not good to use cortisone eye ointments in the eye for long periods because cortisone masks symptoms and could cover up a more serious eye problem. I was careful to place a thin layer on my eye lids only and what a relief! Just using the ointment for a short period of time broke the cycle of itching, rubbing, itching, rubbing.

I resumed Xolair treatments at the end of March 2011. I thought I was doing well. When you live with a condition for a long period of time, you start thinking it is your "norm." I did have short periods of shortness of breath on exertion and just used my inhalers. But, I had to change asthma inhalers as I did not do well on a modified PFT test in August. In September, Workers' Compensation stopped authorizing payment for the drug *again*. We are currently under appeal and another round of legal hearings begins.

I am doing well and my asthma is under control with the Xolair injections. I am afraid to stop them. I have not had a major reaction in the last year. I am not working and do not go out much. I check all areas for latex items. I had no idea just how radically my life would change because of a pair of gloves.

Epilogue.

My frustrations with this allergy prompted me to write this book as one hears little about the allergy and how it affects peoples' lives. As Dr. Richard Edlich wrote in his book *Medicine's Deadly Dust*, "Despite the dramatic life-threatening consequences of [the] latex allergy epidemic, it has not been considered newsworthy...."

My sensitivity to latex and the resultant response have increased with each exposure. Even though I have been very vigilant, I walk into situations I have no control over. My immediate environment is as latex-free as I can make it. When I am shopping, I read all labels and if they don't indicate the material or it doesn't indicate "Ø latex" I don't buy it. That is everything from gardening gloves to coffee mugs. I don't buy any of the cross reactive foods and I wash all vegetables bound with rubber bands. That may be my next crusade—to get produce distributers to stop using rubber bands on asparagus and green onions.

I have to see an allergist on a regular basis and, for now, travel to receive Xolair injections every two weeks. I still have to struggle with Workers' Compensation for medical coverage. As difficult as it is to deal with Worker Compensation issues, I have not given up. My life has been totally consumed by this allergy and by the treatment and lifestyle changes. It has been quite a journey. But most of all, I lost my job as a clinical nurse and teacher.

I will continue to advocate for latex allergy sufferers and have requested the Nevada governor to join in the yearly observance of National Latex Allergy Awareness week which is the first week of October. For further information, I highly recommend the ALAA web site, www.latexallergyresources .org.

Even though new incidences of latex allergy have dropped, because of the reduced use of powdered latex gloves, there still are many among us who have the allergy. I write this book so that others will recognize the struggles of the latex allergic person and to validate those who wrestle with this allergy and the restrictions it causes in their lives. And lastly, to see that they are not forgotten.

I now work to help anyone with a latex allergy and to promote latex safe environments for everyone. I am available for presentations on latex allergy and welcome any invitation.

I have written several articles for the Nevada State Nursing Association regarding my latex allergy, and because of my writing, I have heard from other nurses who have the same problem. I have included their stories in the next chapter.

Part V

Chapter 9

OTHER INDIVIDUAL LATEX ALLERGY EXPERIENCES.

One does not have to be a healthcare professional to acquire a latex allergy. Two of the following stories come from non-healthcare workers: one is an office worker and the other individual acquired the allergy when she was in the second grade. Amazingly, there are many similarities in these stories.

As shown in the following narratives, allergic individuals sometimes tend to downplay the seriousness of the allergy and at times are in denial. The lack of information about latex allergy contributed to the delay in getting diagnosed and to the severity of their reactions. As in Peggy's story, the lack of information caused her to continue to work in hospital departments that were heavily laden with latex products, and getting a proper diagnosis and treatment took several trips to the doctor.

Those afflicted with the allergy had no choice except to leave healthcare, and create their own latex-free environments.

It is evident in their stories how each exposure increased their sensitivity and severity of reactions. Looking back on these stories increases my frustration that we did not know of the seriousness of this allergy sooner.

Denise, dental assistant

Denise was a dental assistant in the mid to late 1980s when the CDC required healthcare workers to use gloves when providing patient care. She worked at her sister's dental office. The first gloves they purchased were vinyl. However, the gloves were ill-fitting, loose, and interfered with detailed dental work. At this time, not knowing the dangers of latex, the office changed to powdered latex gloves, which undoubtedly were more comfortable, better fitting, and allowed the wearer to perform detailed, tactile work.

After a short time, Denise noticed a red itchy rash on her hands that was persistent over the next few years. Eventually she developed a total body rash. Her eyes were itchy, with conjunctival edema, and a constant feeling of fullness.

In 1994, while at work, she rubbed her eye with the sleeve of her latex glove and she had an immediate reaction. Both of her eyes quickly became swollen, red and itchy. That prompted her first trip to the emergency room. From her description of the incident, and her history of dermatitis, she was told she was probably experiencing a latex allergy reaction and was told to stop using latex gloves. Her sister's dental office accommodated her and changed the office gloves to synthetic nitrile.

Later, she decided she wanted to work in the emergency area of healthcare and began attending an Emergency Medical Technician (EMT) class. She followed that class with paramedic training and became a skills instructor for the EMT course. All this time, she was buying her own latex-free gloves and bringing them to her classes.

One day in 1995, when she was on her way to exercise in the local gym she walked through a room filled with latex balloons. Immediately, her eyes began to swell and itch and she broke out in a total body rash. That prompted her second visit to the emergency room. At this time she was told to avoid all latex. She continued to wear non-latex gloves while in her paramedic internship and tried to avoid all latex items. During an EMT lab skills test, she was helping a student perform a skill when Denise inadvertently touched the rubber OB/GYN dummy with bare hands.

This time, she felt tightness in her throat and had difficulty swallowing along with the usual allergic response to her eyes. Thus her third emergency room visit ensued. This time the physician diagnosed her with a Type 1 latex allergy and told her to stay away from all latex and to carry an EpiPen®. Her dream of becoming a paramedic was shattered, and she decided to go back to her sister's dental office where she knew she had support in creating and working in a latex free environment. She also made all the life style changes necessary. No elastic in her clothing, avoidance of balloons and cross reactive fruits—bananas, mangos and kiwi. She carries an EpiPen® everywhere she goes and is on high alert for any latex in her environment. She became pregnant in 1997 and told her physician and the hospital that she had a latex allergy. When it came time to deliver, the hospital did not prepare a latex-safe environment for her. This caused a delay and much frustration. No one could touch her until latex free supplies were found. The situation was quite tense. However, she did delivery a healthy baby boy. Today, she continues strict avoidance, and continues to work in her sister's latex free dental office.

Victoria, RN

Victoria was a dental assistant in the late 1980s. The dental clinic supplied, and she used, powdered latex gloves. Her reactions began in 1989. First, her hands broke out with a rash and itched severely. Eventually, she developed conjunctivitis, and red, itchy, watery eyes. She thought it was the powder causing the reactions. The dental clinic bought different brands of latex gloves looking for one that would not cause Victoria's dermatitis. A new brand would help for a short period of time but the rash eventually returned. She noticed that even when wearing powder-less gloves her symptoms continued. She did not consult with a physician at that time. She did talk to a friendly pharmacist who recommended an eye wash and an over the counter, hydrocortisone cream for her hands. There was no discussion of a possible latex allergy.

In 1991, Victoria decided to leave the dental office and enrolled in a nursing school; from the frying pan into the fire. In the first semester, during her first clinical assignment, she was to bathe a patient. She donned latex gloves and went to work. After dipping her gloved hands in the bathwater she immediately broke out with a severe rash that covered not just her hands but traveled up both arms. Her eyelids swelled and she had difficulty with her vision.

Her instructor quickly responded and opened two Benadryl capsules, placed the powder under her tongue, which stopped the reaction from progressing.

She was required to see an allergist before returning to school. This doctor performed a scratch test using latex serum. She immediately had a 4+ reaction. She was given an adrenaline injection and the allergist diagnosed her with a latex allergy. He gave her latex allergy literature and helped her find a manufacturer of latex-free gloves. He did not give her any further instructions.

She continued her nursing education. The school did not provide any accommodations. While in school she purchased her own latex-free gloves and latex-free tourniquets. She finished school without a problem.

After graduation in 1994, she went to work in a hospital. The hospital still supplied latex gloves in the patient care areas. She had to buy her own latex-free gloves from their central supply department. She began to have bouts of runny nose, watery eyes, and conjunctivitis every day. Even though she used latex- free gloves, she began to suspect other avenues that caused her continued reactions. Since everyone around her used latex gloves, she believed her lab coat carried latex particles. She washed her coat every day. She developed welts on her legs and found that elastic in her undergarments was the cause.

She had reactions after eating food handled by the cafeteria workers wearing latex gloves. She started to bring her own food. She avoided assisting with medical procedures that may involve the use of latex supplies. She did not receive any information regarding latex allergy from her employer. She didn't know what to do. She wanted to be a nurse and never dreamed the reactions would continue.

Her allergist told her the hospital environment was the worst place for her. She was afraid she didn't have any other options. Victoria did not consider filing for Workers' Compensation and after six months she left the hospital. She was offered a position in a medical clinic that provided a latex-safe environment.

She worked there for several years. Eventually, she started her own nurse consulting business.

After a period of time with out reactions Victoria became complacent. She forgot to tell her personal physician she had a latex allergy and had a severe reaction from latex gloves he used during a Pap smear. She had reactions after dental work when she forgot to tell the dentist of her allergy.

Today she is more vigilant about latex in her environment. She chooses clothing that is latex free, uses latex free articles, such as latex-free strip bandages and certain soaps. She carries an EpiPen® and Benadryl, and wears a Medic Alert bracelet. She hasn't had a major reaction for several years, but has to constantly remind herself of the possibilities.

Shari, RN

Shari is an RN and has known about her latex allergy for five years. Her first reaction when wearing latex gloves was severe. She had difficulty breathing, an anaphylactic reaction, and had to go to the emergency room for rescue medications. She avoided latex, but continued to work in hospitals declared latex-safe. However, she has noticed hospitals are again using more latex products.

She is now experiencing an increase in reactions: she reacted to Quark Shoes (made of rubber), keyboard covers, and elastic ear straps on supposedly latex-free isolation masks. She also noticed her face itching after wearing foam earphones.

She tried to be reassigned to a latex-safe environment at the hospital. She says "It is so frustrating to have other nurses' look at me in disbelief when I say I can't use a certain product due to my allergy."

Mary, office worker

Mary, an office worker, noticed rash and itching on her hands after using pens with a rubber grip. Her doctor said she had a dermatitis and to use steroid creams. Her rash cleared. She avoided using rubber grips pens again. She then noticed itching and redness on her hands when driving a car with a steering wheel cover. She also remembers having a strong skin reaction from bandages after having a C-Section. Her skin became bright red with welts. In addition, she remembers getting itchy from the use of Band Aids at home. She was not formally diagnosed with a latex allergy, but she avoids rubber products and she uses non-latex household gloves for washing dishes.

Peggy, RN, MICN

Peggy was an Emergency Room nurse. She had been wearing powdered latex gloves when providing patient care since 1986. She developed dermatitis and cracked dry skin on her hands almost immediately. She thought it was from washing her hands frequently. She used lotions constantly. Eventually, her hands became so ugly she wore the gloves almost all the time to hide her "hamburger hands" from her patients. Her employer was aware and concerned. They would buy different brands of latex gloves. However, they were always powdered. Some gloves were better than others.

Her symptoms persisted and included itchy, watery eyes, and itchy ears. In time, she developed respiratory and gastro intestinal distress.

She saw her first dermatologist around 1994 and was skin tested. She was found to have allergies to many chemicals, including latex. With that information, Peggy was allowed to use nitrile gloves in the Emergency Room when everyone else wore latex gloves.

She was eventually moved to the home health Department in 1996. She found that the "blue gloves" (nitrile) did not cause her hands to break out. She carried and used the blue gloves everywhere she went; she still had reactions from time to time. Everyone else in her department was still wearing powdered latex gloves. Since *she* was using non-latex gloves her doctor implied that she is just anxious and stressed.

With no definite diagnosis linked to powdered latex gloves, Peggy began to train in the operating room (OR). Within six months her respiratory distress increased. By 1998 she was transferred out of the OR and to the out patient department. By this time, more information on latex allergies was available and powdered latex gloves were changed to non-powdered latex gloves.

Incredibly, Peggy still did not have a confirmed diagnosis. Later that year, Peggy had surgery in what was thought to be a latex-safe environment. She developed skin welts and rash at the site of her bandages. Her symptoms progressed to wheezing, itchy and watery eyes, and itchy ears.

She was told by the hospital's risk management department that she needed to see an allergist. Finally, she was diagnosed with combined Type IV and Type I latex allergy.

She filed for Workers' Compensation and went through vocational rehab. She continued to have reactions and could not find a latex-safe work place.

In the spring of 1998, she contacted a lawyer and in 2000 won a settlement from her employer. She also applied for and became eligible for Social Security Disability benefits. She was angry and frustrated that the glove manufactures and CDC did not discover the allergenicity of latex gloves earlier.

Since 2002, she had become super-sensitive. As stated above, it is now known that with each exposure one's sensitivity and severity of reactions increase. Peggy is now allergic to almost all the cross reactive foods including soy. She has reactions even to the least amount of latex in the environment. She also has reactions to food handled by workers who wear latex gloves. She has had many anaphylactic reactions. Her local hospital and emergency care professionals are fully aware of her needs. She carries a respirator mask. She uses this mask in areas that may have latex proteins in the air. She also carries a host of other meds including an EpiPen®.

Pam, electrical engineer

Pam is not a healthcare professional. Currently she is an electrical engineer, technical writer, and book author. Pam is atopic and has seasonal allergies. Her latex allergy started when she was in second grade. Pam wore elastic knee high stockings every day to school. When she developed itchy hives behind her knees her mother changed her socks to ones that had no elastic. She held them up by rolling garter's in the sock. That worked, as the rubber garter did not touch her skin. She also had reactions when wearing rubber household gloves. She began to wear cotton gloves under them.

Later, as a young adult, Pam went to the dentist and while she was there her lip broke out in hives. She thought at first it was a nervous reaction. When she got home, she realized that the dentist and his staff were wearing latex gloves because of the AIDs epidemic.

She was blowing up latex balloons at her daughter's school when her lips began to swell. And then again, while delivering inflated latex balloons in her car she began to wheeze. She opened the windows and quickly delivered the balloons.

She didn't realize that some foods are cross reactive with latex proteins. While eating a banana her ears began to hurt. She didn't think much about it until she told her cousin. He is an oral surgeon. He told her that the banana plant is in the same plant family as the rubber tree, and can cause the same type of latex allergy reactions. He said her eustachian tubes probably swelled and caused the ear pain. She then noticed she would break out in hives after eating melons; honeydew, cantaloupe and watermelon. Once after eating a plum her voice changed. She stated her voice went down 2 octaves. She then realized her vocal cords must be swollen.

She finally went to see an allergist and had extensive testing. She had many reactive skin tests. Her allergist said her back "lit up like a Christmas tree." Now she carries an EpiPen® and avoids all the cross-reactive foods. She discovered if she eats small amounts of the forbidden fruits she does not have a reaction.

Yet after all that, Pam downplayed her allergic status to rubber when she went to an orthodontist for braces. She told the dentist that her allergy was "not that bad." Unfortunately, within 24 hours of rubber bands on her braces, her mouth swelled. She took Benadryl and had all the rubber bands changed to vinyl. She now avoids all latex products.

Traci, RN, MSN

In 1990, while working in the labor and delivery department using powdered latex gloves, Traci developed dermatitis on her hands. She wasn't sure what was causing the rash until she read an article in the California Nursing Association newsletter. It stated there have been reports of allergic contact dermatitis related to the powder used in latex gloves. She began treating the rash with cortisone creams. She noticed the rash would disappear when she was away from work. In 1992, her employer started using non-powdered latex gloves. Her dermatitis cleared.

In 1994, she moved to another city and was working in labor and delivery in a local hospital. The rash returned in intensity this time with facial redness, watery eyes and wheezing. She suspected she had a latex allergy but did not have a definite diagnosis. Two years later, while working in a Utah hospital, she was using non-latex nitrile gloves. However, other staff members in the labor and delivery department wore latex gloves. She was told to wear latex over the nitrile gloves when working with the labor and delivery patients as latex was a better barrier against blood-borne pathogens.

This time she had her first anaphylactic reaction. She was sent to ER and treated. She was told to follow up with an allergist. He performed skin tests using a latex glove soaked in saline solution and taped a piece of glove to her skin. She had an anaphylactic reaction in his office. This allergist finally diagnosed her with a latex allergy.

When she returned to work she was moved to the post partum department. It was thought she would have less latex exposure in that department. She also decided to finish her bachelor's degree and work towards a post graduate degree in order to teach nursing. She moved to Las Vegas in 2000 and again began working in the labor delivery department of a local hospital. She was having minor reactions and was managing them with her prescribed medication. While assisting with a C-Section at the hospital, Traci began to wheeze and her face became crimson. She was ordered out of the surgical suite and sent to ER in an anaphylactic state. That was her last hospital assignment. She was placed on a medication regime of Benadryl, Pepcid, and Claritin, and was given an EpiPen®.

She completed her post graduate degree and began teaching in a registered nurse program. She continued to have manageable reactions and finally became a nursing lab instructor at a local college. The lab was deemed latex safe. Traci was cautious about latex supplies being donated to the school from other facilities. She made sure her own equipment was latex free. During one of her lab sessions the students brought in their own blood pressure cuffs. The cuffs had a latex bladder and latex hand pump. Traci began to wheeze and went into a full anaphylactic reaction. Paramedics were called and she was admitted to the hospital.

The university changed her full time position to adjunct. She has not been given any teaching assignments. She is applying for disability through her employer. Traci had become very hypersensitive to latex anywhere in her environment. She has had reactions in grocery stores and even department stores. She avoids places that use latex balloons. She calls restaurants checking for use of latex gloves. Her four-year-old daughter has also been diagnosed with a latex allergy when she had a reaction while wearing a Band Aid.

APPENDIX
Time line for Glove History in Health Care

1890   First time rubber gloves used in surgery.

1920   Acceptance of sterile gloves, gowns and mask as routine practice in surgery

1933   First reported hand dermatitis from rubber gloves

1960   Disposable latex gloves become available. Still only used in surgery and sterile procedures

1981   First Reported case of AIDS

1982   Hepatitis B becomes a national concern

1983   CDC recommends latex glove use; Blood and Body Fluids Precautions (for suspected Hepatitis B infections-HIV wasn't identified yet)

1984   HIV virus identified and now begins to be a national concern

1985   CDC changes Blood and Body Fluids Precautions to Universal Blood and Body Fluid Precautions (now including anyone suspected of HIV infections)

1987   Universal Blood and Body Fluid Precautions changed to Standard Precautions. Gloves are to be worn for any contact with blood or body fluids. In addition, gowns, masks, and protective eye wear had to be worn. Now, all patients are to be treated as having an infectious disease.

1988   OSHA joins CDC in mandating Standard Precautions

1991   Government begins educating about HIV

1993   Isolated reports of hand dermatitis and illnesses among healthcare workers

1997   First NIOSH bulletin on latex allergy published regarding wearing latex gloves. Information on latex allergy finally becoming available

1998   FDA banishes labeling latex gloves (non-hypoallergenic)

REFERENCES

American College of Allergy, Asthma, and Immunology (ACAAI), & American Academy of Allergy, Asthma, and Immunology (AAAAI) (1997). Joint statement concerning the use of powdered and non-powdered natural rubber latex gloves. Annals of Allergy, Asthma, and Immunology, 79(6), 487.

American Latex Allergy Association (ALAA)
www.latexallergyresources.org

Amr, S. & Suk W.A. (2004). Latex allergy and occupational asthma in health care workers: Adverse outcomes. Environmental Health Perspectives, 112 (3), March 2004

Antiseptic and Aseptic Techniques are Developed. Retrieved from www. Bookrags.com/research/antiseptic-and-aseptic-techniques-a-scit-051234

Apocynaceae: The periwinkle family. Retrieved from: http://theseedsite.co. uk/apocynaceae.html

Beezhold, D. H., Reschke, J. E., Allen, J.H., Kostyal, D. A. & Sussman, G. L. (2000). Latex protein: A hidden food allergen? Allergy and Asthma Proceedings Sept-Oct 21 (5), 301-6.

Center for Disease Control (CDC) www.cdc.gov/hiv/topics/surveillance/resources/slides/in dex.htm

Goodyear, Charles. Story. Retrieved from www.goodyear.com/corporate/history/history_story.html

Goodyear, Charles. Retrieved from www.nndb.com/people/411/000050261

Macintosh, Charles. Retrieved from www.whonamedit.com/doctor.cfm/ 2089.html

Craig, Maggie, "The History of Surgical Gloves." Retrieved from www.ehow.com/about6572251_history-surgical-gloves.html

DeLeo, V. A. (2006). Contact allergen of the year: p- Phenylenediamine. Dermatitis 2006, 17(2), 53-55

Downing, J.G. (1933) Dermatitis from rubber gloves. New England Journal of Medicine 139:1223. Retrieved from http://www.immune.com/rub ber/rubber_gloves.html

Duffield, L.D. (1998) Latex allergy: Everyone's concern. Journal of the Michigan Dental Association, June 1998. Retrieved from www.latex allergylinks.org/MDA.html

Dunbrook, R. F. (1996). Rubber. Colliers Encyclopedia, CD-Rom, Vol 20, 02-28-1996. Retrieved from www.slac.com/tree/research/styrene/rubber.html

Edlich, R. F. (1997). Medicine's deadly dust.(pp 77-87). Vandamere Press: Arlington, VA.

Ferguson, L. K., and Sholtis, L.A. (1959). Eliason's surgical nursing (11th ed). Operating room nursing, .Lippincott: Philadelphia .

Finny, D. (2006) Mayan Games Retrieved from www.greatdreams.com/mayan/mayangames.htm

Grier, T. (2009). Latex Allergy: Latex cross reactive foods. Retrieved from American Latex Allergy Association website www.latexallergyresources.org

Groce, D. F.(1996). Cotton, nylon, lycra, spandex, and allergies. Latex Allergy News .Retrieved October 2011, from latexallergyresources.org

History of AIDS in America, 1980, 1990, 2000. Retrieved from www.avert.org/aids-history-america.htm

History of Latex Gloves: Part 2. William Stewart Halsted, The father of "safe" surgery. Retrieved from www.palmflex.com/blog?tag=rubber-gloves

History of Latex Gloves: Part 3. Neil Tillotson, The wizard of Dixville Notch. Retrieved from www.palmflex.com/blog?tag=rubber-gloves

HIV/AIDS statistics and surveillance. Basic statistics, Retrieved from www.cdc.gov/hiv/topics/surveillance/basic.htm

HIV in the United States. Retrieved from www.cdc.gov/hiv/surveillance/factsheets.htm

Huether, S.E. & McCance, K.L. (2008) Understanding Pathophysiology (4th ed.) Chapter 7. St Louis, Mosby.

Jacobs, S.E. & Steele, T. (2006) Allergic contact dermatitis: Early recognition and diagnosis of important allergies. Dermatology Nursing (2006) 18 (5), 443-439.

Latex Allergy; Cleveland Clinic (1995-2009). Retrieved July 22, 2009 from www.myclevelandclinic.org/disorders/Latex_Allergy/hic_Latex_Allerg y.aspx

Lackman, M. Latex or Lycra: The facts behind the fibers. Retrieved October 16, 2011 from www.OrganicClothing.blogs.com

Lane, Alice, History of surgical attire from the suit to the sterile scrubs of today. Retrieved from zinearticles.com/?expert=alicelane

Medical Exam Gloves www.medicalexamgloves.com/latex/manufacturing_process.html

Miller, J.T., Rahimi, S.Y., Lee, M. History of Infection Control and its Contributions to the Development and Success of Brain Tumor Operations (2005). American Association of Neurological Surgeons 18 (4),1-5. Retrieved from www.medscape.com/viewarticle/503947

MMWR -Vol.38, No.S-6 (1989). Guidelines for prevention of transmission of human immunodeficiency virus and Hepatitis B virus to health-care and public safety workers. Retrieved from www.cdc.gov/mmwr.mmwrsch.htm

More, D. (2009). What is the latex-food syndrome? Retrieved from www.allergies.about.com/od/medicationallergies/alatexfood.html

Muller, B.A., Steelman, V.M., Hartley, P.G., and Casale, T. B.(1998). An approach to managing latex allergy in the health care worker. *Journal of Environmental Health*, Vol. 61, Issue 1.

National Legal Resource and Strategy Center for HIV Advocacy www.hivlawandpolicy.org

National Institute for Occupational Safety and Health, "Preventing Allergic Reactions to Natural Rubber Latex in the Workplace (1997)." NIOSH Publication No. 97-135. Cincinnati, OH.

Nelson, R. T. (2011). AIDS deaths worldwide declining, New infection leveling off.. Retrieved from www.fairwarning.org/2011/11/aids-deaths-worldwide-declining

Nettis, E., Assinnato, G., Ferranini, A. and Tursi, A. (2002). Type 1 allergy to natural rubber latex and type iv allergy to rubber chemicals in health care worker. *Clinical Experience Allergy*, Mar 32(3)441-7.

Nightingale, F.(1860). Notes on Nursing. An unabridged republication as published by D. Appleton and Company (1860) by Dover Publications Inc. © 1969.

Organic Clothing: Latex or Lycra? : Facts behind the fibers. Retrieved from organicclothing.blogs.com/my_weblog/2006/08/latex_or lycra_jtml

Occupational Safety and Health Administration . "Occupational Exposure to Bloodborne Pathogens. Section 3 - III.
Events leading to final standard (1991)." Retrieved from
www.osha.gov/pls/oshaweb/owadisp.show_document?p_table=
PREAMBLES&p_id=805

Occupational Safety and Health Administration. "Potential for sensitization and possible allergic reaction to natural rubber latex gloves and other natural rubber products." *Safety and Health Bulletin. SHIB 01-28-2008.* Retrieved from
www.osha.gov/dts/shib/shib012808.html

Phillips, V.L.D. Phil, Goodrich, M. A., and Sullivan, T.J.(1999). Health-care worker disability due to latex allergy and asthma: A cost analysis. *American Journal of Public Health, Vol.89,No 7.*

Price, A.L.(1959). *The Art, Science and Spirit of Nursing* (2nd ed.). W.B. Saunders Company: Philadelphia

Shomon, M. (2006) *Understanding the Immune System.* Retrieved from throid.about.com/library/immune/blimm19.htm?p=1   Pacific Northwest Foundation,(2005). *The Complete Guide to Latex Allergy,* Portland, OR.

Hancock, Thomas. Retrieved from http://www.bouncing-balls.com/time line/people/nr_hancock.html

Witt, S.F. (1999). Potential for allergy to natural rubber latex gloves and other natural rubber products. *Technical Information   Bulletin.* OSHA, Washington DC Retrieved from www.latexallergylinks. org/LA-TIB.html

Wood, D.A. (2008). Latex Gloves Becoming History. *Nursing Spectrum/NurseWeek.* Retrieved from http://news.nurse.com/apps/ pbcs.dll/article?AID=/20080324/OR02/ 303250001

INDEX

diarrhea, 48
disability
    codes and ratings, 26
    insurance, 56
    See also California State Disability Division
disposable patient care supplies, 39-41
Downing, J.G., xii, 33-34
Doxipen, 22

E
Edlich, Richard F., 12, 43, 46, 49, 67
EKG monitoring pads, 52
ELISA/ACT program, 11
Emergency Room visits, 15, 70, 73-74
employment issues
    career change, 28, 52-55
employer's inability to accommodate, 56, 63-64
    forced retirement, 101
    job duty reassignments, 21, 55-56
    medical leaves of absence, 11, 21, 56, 63
    Post-diagnosis, 21-28
    work release, 15, 17, 20
EpiPen®, 77
erythema, 48
eye symptoms
    cortisone eye ointments, 11, 66
eye drops usage, 9, 13, 52
    NIOSH alert bulletin, 13-14
    puffy/red/itchy/watery, 9-10, 15, 48, 53, 61, 65, 70-71, 75
    swelling, 48

F
flu pandemic (1918), 37
food allergies
    author's experiences with, 11-12, 23-24, 52, 61

hepatitis B (HBV)
  and glove mandate, 1, 4-5
  rise of, xi
  vaccination program proposal by CDC, 4
heterosexual activity, and spread of HIV virus, 2
Hevea brasiliensis tree, 31, 48
histamine, 12, 22, 47, 62
HIV (Human Immunodeficiency Virus)
  and blood transfusions, 2
  confidentiality laws, 5-7
  emergence of, xi
  etiology of, 2-3
  and routine glove use, 4-6
  written consent for antibody testing, 6
  See also AIDS (Acquired Immunodeficiency Syndrome)
hives, 12-13, 75-76
hotel rooms, 60-61
Hudson, Rock, 2
Hydroxyzine (Vistaril), 22, 58
Hypersensitivity. *See* allergic (hypersensitivity) response
hypnosis, 11
hypoallergenic, use of term, 12, 34
hypotension, 48

I

IBT latex specific IgE panel blood tests, 15-16
IgE allergic asthma, 62
IgE antibodies, 47
IgE mediated latex allergy
  blood test for, 15, 16
  cause of, 14
  and cross-reactivity/fruit syndrome, 48-50
IgE antibodies, 47
  See also allergic (hypersensitivity) response
immune system

M

sick building syndrome, 12
See also photographs of symptoms
respiratory tract, 12, 44, 47-48, 53, 60, 64
See also asthma; bronchial symptoms
restaurants, and latex glove use, 58-61
retirement, forced into, 101
rhinitis, 48
right to work states, 57
Risk Management Company, 25-26
rubber, allergenic properties of, 33-34
See also headings at latex
rubber bands, 67
rubber trees, 29-31, 76

S
Saylor, John, 20-22, 25-26, 52, 54, 62, 65
Seiberling, Frank, 31
Semmelweis, Ignaz, 35
sick building syndrome, 12
Simian Immunodeficiency Virus (SIV), 2
skin reactions. *See* dermatitis symptoms; photographs of symptoms
Spandex, 16-18, 22, 58
Standard Precautions (CDC/OSHA), xi, 5
steam sterilization, 36
sterilization practices, 38, 40
stomach cramps, 48
surgical asepsis, 38
surgical attire and gloves, 36-41
surgical greens, 37-38
Sutter Hospital, 20
swimsuits. *See* bathing suits
symptoms, author's experiences with. *See* photographs of symptoms; specific symptoms
systemic, anaphylactic allergic reactions, 47

BIOGRAPHY

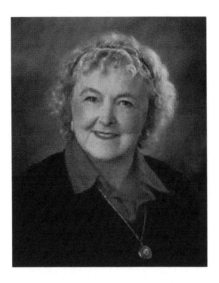

Margaret Konieczny is a Registered Nurse. She graduated in 1964 from Holy Cross School of Nursing in South Bend, Indiana. In 2002 she earned her Masters of Nursing Degree at California State University, Dominguez Hills.

She has enjoyed a long extensive career in hospital nursing. She started her career at Los Angeles County Medical Center in the fall of 1964. She continued her career at Kaiser Hospital in Harbor City, CA. St. Joseph's Hospital in Phoenix, AZ. and O'Connor Hospital in San Jose, CA. She became employed at Barton Memorial Hospital in South Lake Tahoe in 1975. The HIV crisis began while she was at Barton; where she was diagnosed with a Type IV and Type I latex allergy in 1998. She left hospital nursing and began teaching nursing at Western Nevada Community College in 2002.

She continued to have latex exposures and she experienced a forced retirement in 2010. Margaret presently holds a current Nevada nursing license and is a member of the nurse practice advisory board of the Nevada

State Board of Nursing. She is an active member of the American Latex Allergy Association and will speak to anyone who is interested in hearing the latex story. She is currently a successful author of a children's book, *Ten Finger Prints in the Butter* and has been published in the Nevada State Nursing Association newsletter.

Find out more at:
www.latexallergystories.com/
www.mynursingstories.com/

Made in the USA
Columbia, SC
15 September 2021